Making Tuberculosis History

Making Tuberculosis History

Community-based Solutions for Millions

BRAC Health Program

Md. Akramul Islam
Maria A. May
Faruque Ahmed
Richard A. Cash
Jalaluddin Ahmed

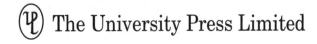 The University Press Limited

9030 0000 143 210

The University Press Limited
Red Crescent House
61 Motijheel C/A, P. O. Box 2611
Dhaka 1000, Bangladesh
Fax : (88 02) 9565443
E-mail: upl@bangla.net, upl@btcl.net.bd
Website: www.uplbooks.com.bd

First published, 2011

Copyright © The University Press Limited, 2011

Cover design by Shajedur Rahman, BRAC

Photo Credits: All photos from BRAC archive. Photographs 7, 9, 15 and 16 on pages 136, 137 and 140 by Shehzad Noorani/BRAC.

ISBN 978 984 506 039 4

Published by Mohiuddin Ahmed, The University Press Limited, Dhaka. Book design by Ashim K. Biswas and produced by Abarton, 354 Dilu Road, Moghbazar. Printed at the Akota Offset Press, 119 Fakirapool, Dhaka, Bangladesh.

Contents

List of Tables and Figures

Tables

Figures

Selected Photographs of BRAC's TB Program

Acronyms and Translations

Af	Afghani (currency of Afghanistan)
ART	Antiretroviral therapy
BGMEA	Bangladesh Garments Manufacturers and Exporters Association
BPHS	Basic package of health services (Afghanistan Ministry of Health)
(TB) CAP	TB Control Assistance Program (USAID)
CCM	Country coordinating mechanism
CIDA	Canadian International Development Agency
DFID	Department for International Development (United Kingdom)
DOTS	Directly observed therapy, short-course
FIDELIS	Fund for Innovative DOTS Expansion through Local Initiatives to Stop TB
KAP	Knowledge, attitudes, and practices
LTFU	Lost to follow up
MDR TB	Multidrug resistant TB
NATAB	National Anti-Tuberculosis Association of Bangladesh
NGO	Non-governmental organization
NTP	National Tuberculosis Program
ORT	Oral rehydration therapy
OTEP	Oral therapy extension program (BRAC)
RED	Research and evaluation division (BRAC)
RIT	Research Institute of TB of Japan
SIDA	Swedish International Development Agency
TB	Tuberculosis

Tk	Taka (currency of Bangladesh)
USAID	United States Agency for International Development
USD	United States' Dollar
WHO	World Health Organization
XDR TB	Extremely drug resistant TB

English translations of Bangla words and phrases

Gur	Unrefined brown sugar
Hartal	Strike and/or demonstration as political protest
Jokkha	Colloquial word for tuberculosis
Jumma	Friday prayer
Matbor	Local elite
Samity	Village collective
Shasthya kormi	(BRAC) health worker
Shasthya shebika	(BRAC) female health volunteer
Shasthya shebok	(BRAC) male health volunteer
Shushasthya	(BRAC) health center
Thana or upazila	Sub-district (483 in total)

Foreword

Holistic or integrated programming requires precision and careful attention to detail. For each intervention, BRAC has developed a disciplined process of designing, evaluating, refining, scaling and evolving the model to ensure its continuous relevance and effectiveness. Our tuberculosis program is an example of what this process can engender. In 1984, we began to pilot ways to bring services typically offered only in urban health facilities to the villages of Bangladesh. We ensured that patients could get sputum testing without leaving the village. In fact, the entire treatment could be provided at the village as well, under the supervision of a local woman trained as a community health volunteer. This model took us some years to evaluate and refine; we knew that if we wanted to take it to national scale, we needed all the components—incentives, training, supervision, quality control—aligned before we started to expand. We would also need to find synergies, within BRAC's own programs and with others, like the National Tuberculosis Program of the government.

Common wisdom is that a program has to choose between scale and quality; one cannot do both. At BRAC, we have continuously and successfully challenged this notion. With TB control as well, we wanted to show that a large program could achieve good results if it was well designed and managed. Reflecting on the past 27 years, I think BRAC has done just that. Without compromising the high cure rate, we've gone from a pilot of a few hundred cases to treating close to 100,000 annually. A leader in the national public-private partnership, BRAC also manages the efforts of over 40 other NGOs participating in TB control in Bangladesh. If programs are designed to provide quality at scale, they can.

These principles have relevance beyond Bangladesh. In 2002, BRAC began to work internationally. Once we started working in Afghanistan, it didn't take long to see that in many ways, poor people there faced the same problems as the poor of Bangladesh: limited physical and operational access to important services like health and shortages of trained personnel. As we set up our microfinance, education, and community health volunteer programs, we developed the confidence and ambition to push ourselves to expand our mission more globally. Certainly new contexts provide new challenges, but a strong principled and a tested approach guided us through the processes of adaptation and innovation. Our experiences with TB control in Afghanistan and Uganda provides some ideas of these experiences.

South-South partnerships offer an opportunity for learning and change, a chance to redefine common wisdom, and a challenge to make scale imperative to development work. In too many countries around the world, TB remains a critical health challenge. I hope that this story inspires its readers and provides them with examples of how the BRAC model may be translated into their own programs and environments.

Sir Fazle Hasan Abed KCMG
Founder and Chairperson

Acknowledgements

The motivation for developing this book was a reflection on the accomplishments that BRAC has had in its TB program over the past 27 years. The authors humbly acknowledge that they are simply representing the stories of others, of the implementers and supporters who have taken the program from a small pilot and grown it into a model that covers millions. Not surprisingly, the list of those to recognize is long, but we have tried to at least give credit to all those who have made significant contributions.

The Ministry of Health and Family Welfare of Bangladesh and the National Tuberculosis Program have been supporting our program since the 1980s. We are indebted for the many contributions that they have made and are quite grateful for how they have chosen to strengthen the partnership over time. In recent years, the efforts of the Bangladesh Country Coordinating Mechanism to ensure resources for TB control activities in Bangladesh have also been critical for our ability to scale. We would like to thank Khondokar Md. Shefyetullah (Directorate General of Health Services), Motiuddin Ahmed (Directorate General of Health Services), and Md. Ashaque Husain (National Tuberculosis Program) for their commitment to TB control and leadership in ensuring that services reach communities across the country.

In recent years, we've also had the opportunity to contribute to the efforts of the Afghanistan Ministry of Public Health to develop the country's health system and support the introduction of community-based TB control. We appreciate the contributions made by the Afghanistan Country Coordinating Mechanism to mobilize resources for these activities.

Many individuals made tremendous contributions to the development of this book and the program. There are a few to whom we would like to give special recognition. Nobukatsu Ishikawa (Research Institute of Tuberculosis, Japan) has provided personal and institutional support since program's beginnings in 1984. He has been with the program every step of the way, sharing his wealth of expertise and encouraging us with humor and enthusiasm. Our former colleague, Mushtaque Chowdhury (Rockefeller Foundation), ensured that from our early activities, we had a research lens, and he was the first to share the BRAC experiences in TB through international publications. He has been a vigorous advocate of the community model and provided rigorous evidence through his research on how the program could be improved over time.

During the initial pilot (1984-1990), the late Md. Aminul Alam (BRAC), Md. Shirajul Islam (National TB Program), and Sakhawat Hussain (NATAB) worked tirelessly to implement and evaluate TB control activities in the communities of Manikganj. During the early 1990s, when BRAC scaled up its pilot to 10 sub-districts and entered a formal partnership with the government for TB control, several individuals played an instrumental role in making these activities successful, notably our former colleague Sadia Chowdhury (World Bank), A.K. Md. Ahsan Ali and Jalal Uddin Ahmed (National Tuberculosis Program), and Lisa Parkkali (World Health Organization). Fazlul Karim (BRAC) began to support the TB program during this time and remains an important source of monitoring and research to ensure that the program continuously improves.

Scale up, particularly of the magnitude that BRAC envisioned, can only be achieved with great leadership and management. BRAC benefited from the dedication and relentless efforts of Mahabub Hossain, Shib Narayan Kairy, Imran Matin, Kaosar Afsana, and the late Md. Aminul Alam, and they deserve particular thanks for their contributions and leadership. Sukhendra K. Sarkar (BRAC) deserves thanks for his contributions in supporting the internal control of the program as it grew. We also have great appreciation for the commitment and efforts of Mahfuza Rifat, who has provided significant leadership with the TB program from 2004. Mrinal Kanti Biswas, Nasrin Ara Begum, Milan Kanti Barua, Bivakar Roy, Mohamed Shahjahan, Shayla Islam and all members of the BRAC TB program have enabled the program to grow quickly and efficiently.

The BRAC TB program also enjoys the support of many other departments and institutions that have been critical to its effectiveness. In particular, BRAC's Research and Evaluation Division (RED), the Management Information System (MIS), and the Finance and

Accounts Department support in our everyday operations and generously assisted us throughout the book-writing process.

The World Health Organization (WHO) has provided significant technical support in our activities. Our other partners, including the National Anti-TB Association of Bangladesh and the Damien Foundation, make significant contributions to TB control in Bangladesh, and we benefit greatly from their experience and willingness to share. The Urban Primary Health Care Project and the Bangladesh Garment Manufacturers' and Exporters' Association are also critical partners for TB control. We also appreciate the city corporation authorities, Bangladesh Medical Association, professional bodies, academic institutions, and prison authorities that support and participate in BRAC's TB control activities.

Several international institutions are instrumental in helping us improve our programs. In particular, we are appreciative of the Research Institute of Tuberculosis of Japan and the International Union against Tuberculosis and Lung Disease.

Funding from the Global Fund to Fight AIDS, TB, and Malaria has transformed TB control in Bangladesh, enabling activities to reach their current scale. Other donors we'd like to acknowledge for current or historical support include: the United Kingdom's Department for International Development, the Canadian International Development Agency, the Fund for Innovative Expansion through Local Initiatives to Stop TB (FIDELIS) through the International Union against TB and Lung Disease, the European Union, the Swedish International Development Agency, Oxfam Novib, United States' Agency for International Development, the Australian Government Overseas Aid Program (AusAID), and the United Nations' Children's Fund.

Sharmin Ferdous (BRAC) assisted extensively in the research and document gathering that this book entailed. Taufiqur Rahman (BRAC) and Fazlul Hoque (BRAC) provided guidance in the development of Chapter 8 on Afghanistan. Reflections on BRAC's TB control efforts in Uganda certainly benefited from discussions with Khondaker Ariful Islam (BRAC). BRAC's Communications Department kindly provided support and input on graphics and other aspects of book development. The data gathered in Laura Reichenbach's and Shafiun Nahin Shimul's (International Center for Diarrheal Disease Research, Bangladesh) comprehensive assessment of the community health volunteer programs in several countries greatly informed Chapter 6. Khurshid Alam Hyder (WHO), Marijke Becx (formerly WHO), Vikarunnessa Begum (WHO), Abdul Hamid Salim (KNCV Tuberculosis Foundation, formerly Damien Foundation), and Aung Kya Jai (Damien Foundation) also provided guidance on historical sections.

Mushtaque Chowdhury (Rockefeller Foundation), Joseph Rhatigan (Brigham and Women's Hospital), Nobukatsu Ishikawa (Research Institute of Tuberculosis, Japan) Masud Ahmed (BRAC), Fazlul Karim (BRAC), I.D. Rusen (International Union against TB and Lung Disease), and Donald Enarson (International Union against TB and Lung Disease) provided valuable commentary on drafts. A few additional friends and colleagues were kind enough to permit us to interview them in the development of this book. We appreciate their time and insight; readers will find many of their comments in the text.

In keeping with BRAC's mission, we would like to acknowledge that at the heart of the program are the field workers and the communities: our staff and volunteers (shasthya shebikas) actively implement BRAC's mission daily; it is their accomplishments that we are truly celebrating on these pages. It is exciting to see BRAC's TB program expanding abroad and touching more lives.

Sir Fazle Hasan Abed (BRAC) had an ambitious dream for the TB program from its inception. We are most indebted for his continuous inspiration and reminder to keep improving.

Chapter 1

Introduction: The Scale Imperative

Located on the 16th floor of a nondescript building on Mohakhali Avenue in Dhaka, the head office of BRAC's health program resembles a crowded newsroom. The bright colors of women dressed in *salwar kameez* and *sarees* and the clinking sounds of tea cups on the desks exude an unmistakably Bengali character. Often there are power outages or cuts in the internet, and the staff gather in small groups, waiting for them to be restored while discussing plans instead of sending emails. They nod and take notes in the blue journals that are distributed to all staff each calendar year. To the north lies Korail, a bustling slum settlement perched on a manmade island. Watching individuals shuttle back and forth to the main road in small boats, one observes the daily struggles that many face to survive and the scale of the challenges yet to overcome.

Five times a day, there are prayer calls in the distance from the neighborhood mosques. Some staff members quietly excuse themselves for prayer and find a quiet space in one of the conference rooms or hallways to lay out their prayer rugs. Fridays, the Muslim day of *jumma* (Friday prayer), is a consistent weekend but on Saturdays many staff can be found in the office, hard at work on their responsibilities that were put off during the week, with the many unavoidable meetings with non-governmental organization (NGO) partners, government staff, donors, and others that pull them away from program and management activities. For the world's largest NGO, this is business as usual. Born in the wake of Bangladesh's war for independence from Pakistan, as 10 million refugees who had been displaced to India returned to a homeland devastated by a recent cyclone and civil war, BRAC has grown with the nation, under the leadership of Bangladeshis, and operates large-scale programs in the context of a developing country, with all the challenges and opportunities that it affords. While it has been touched by some of the world's most prestigious universities and institutions, it remains proudly and distinctly Bengali in its philosophy and its practices, able to function in the midst of unavoidable challenges that the developing country environment so often presents.

Despite after forty years of furiously paced work, there is still a daily sense that there are needs that must be met and resources that must be stretched as far as humanly possible. The central office of 2,100 staff members oversees an army of 46,000 field staff, 65,000 teachers, and 89,000 community health volunteers, serving over 110 million Bangladeshis. The number of communities it serves internationally continues to grow. Already it is one of the largest NGOs in Afghanistan and Uganda.

Scale is at the core of BRAC's work. Its founder, Sir Fazle Hasan Abed, is often quoted as saying, "small is beautiful, but big is necessary." In Bangladesh, BRAC pilots programs at the *upazila* (sub-district) level, with a population of 250,000, and thinks of scale in terms of in millions. Since its program in the 1980s to combat death from diarrheal diseases, BRAC's idea of scale has increasingly implied national level coverage. Consequently, BRAC's health programs are designed with careful attention to local resources and sustainability.

There are a number of organizations hard at work to alleviate poverty and improve health around the world, but none has reached the scale of BRAC's activity. In conversations about "universal access" or "health for all," the need for scaling up is clear. Governments and private partners alike must adopt models that can be scaled and develop the management systems to maintain them. Certainly these tasks present challenges, but BRAC's success in Bangladesh and other countries creates a compelling case that it is far from impossible. For all the importance of local relevance, BRAC has found that, fundamentally, the condition of poverty is characterized by lack of access to critical services and products, limited resources, and significant vulnerability to outside forces. BRAC's package of education, microfinance, agriculture, income generation, and health, when adapted and delivered by local staff and communities, appears to transfer across a variety of sociopolitical settings and maintain its ability to spread like wildfire. Even in the complex environment of urban areas, BRAC continues to push its programs to cover large populations, through partnerships with private providers, NGOs, and government. "Taking health to the people" can take many forms; BRAC's dedication to its mission forces flexibility in its strategies.

At its core, BRAC is an implementing agency—its staff is most comfortable in the field, working alongside community members. While this singular focus has led to strong results in the field, there has often been an underinvestment in documentation and reflection. Geographic scale may be BRAC's comfort area, but by disseminating its knowledge and practices to other implementers and policy-makers, its impact might be even greater. In the early 1990s, the book *A Simple Solution* was written cataloging BRAC's activities in community-based education and training on treating diarrheal disease with a homemade oral rehydration therapy (ORT). In its oral therapy extension program (OTEP) of the 1980s, BRAC taught 12 million mothers and child caretakers how to prepare and use ORT. Even today, Bangladesh has the highest use rate of ORT in the world. Telling the story opened up the possibility of scaling up health programs to many who were not directly part of the Bangladesh experience. In 2005, under the editorial leadership of Jon Rohde, another book on BRAC's programs emerged. Along with the oral rehydration extension program, it described the experiences of several other health programs, along with reflections on BRAC's overarching approach to learning and integration of research in program activities (Rohde, 2005).

The experience with oral rehydration set the wheels in motion for BRAC's large-scale approach to community health. Heartened by the scale achieved in its OTEP program, in the 1980s BRAC began looking for other public health challenges for it to tackle at a similar scale. It observed that for many rural villagers, tuberculosis (TB) was a death sentence, despite the existence of an effective 12-month course of medications. Upon bringing medicines to the villagers, BRAC realized that the challenge was more complex: patients began to feel better quickly and stopped taking the medications long before their TB was cured. Adherence was just one challenge to tackle; before thinking about scale, BRAC also had to account for the challenges of addressing a disease that required microscopic diagnosis, carried a degree of stigmatization in the community, and could present side effects that community health volunteers would be unable to treat. It needed to attack the processes of scaling up with the same attention to detail and investments in building the structure that the program wouldn't outgrow. Twenty-seven years later, BRAC's TB program, in essence, is an example of a program that achieves very high levels of adherence for a low cost, with limited resources, and at a large scale. We hope that these lessons can be instructive to others engaged in TB control. As many of these principles are not exclusive to TB, we challenge ourselves and our readers to think about the broader applicability of these experiences to other conditions.

From its inception, BRAC's TB control program has involved leadership and support from other partners locally and abroad. In tandem with BRAC's own growth, the National Tuberculosis Program expanded free treatment nationally, with over 158,000 patients receiving treatment from its facilities or partners annually in 2010 (NTP, 2011). These achievements are due to the activities of individual institutions, but also processes that link the activities of over 40 diverse partners. As one of the National Tuberculosis Program's initial NGO partners, BRAC is the largest implementer and a leader in the overall effort. We explore how the partnership has enabled BRAC's scale and how it will help BRAC best adjust its strategies to meet emerging challenges of TB control in Bangladesh.

From its humble beginnings in 1984, we present the whole history of BRAC's work in TB to guide others interested in solving the problem of scaling up health programs and sustaining them. Details of the field-level activities, management system, strategies and even finances of the program are presented to provide a thorough, multi-level description of the program. Some readers might find the level of detail captured here exhaustive (or exhausting); decades of implementation has proven that careful attention to detail is essential, whether the context is flood-prone villages of Bangladesh, mountainous provinces of Afghanistan, or the lakes shores of Uganda.

Over the years, BRAC has carefully changed elements of the TB program to tailor it precisely to the Bangladeshi rural and urban contexts. We have attempted here to deconstruct the program to enable others to apply the *principles*, rather than the activity set itself, in ways that are best adapted to their own setting. Selection of practitioners, provision of adequate management, appropriate monitoring and evaluation, and alignment of incentives are universal challenges in health delivery. Additionally, organizations that hope to sustain their value must not only create a program with these criteria, but also maintain the flexibility to identify changes and respond in a timely fashion without compromising the quality of their programming.

As BRAC expands its health programs within Afghanistan, Pakistan, Haiti, Uganda, Tanzania, Sierra Leone, and, Liberia, our interest in codifying these principles is no longer simply academic or altruistic. Our programs in a few African countries must grapple with the best strategies to address HIV, a disease which to date has fortunately remained quite limited in Bangladesh. The growing focus internationally on the burden of chronic conditions and maternal health likely indicates greater attention to previously neglected conditions and an immediate demand for creating and scaling effective programs. The shift in focus may mean that programs working on malaria, TB and HIV must do more with less or demonstrate more convincingly the value of their programs. Exploiting economies of scale and leveraging community-based programs will be essential.

1.1 Organization of the book

The book is divided into three parts: historical context; current Bangladesh TB control program; and expansion. The next three chapters recount BRAC's earliest health programs and the pilot and scale up on BRAC's tuberculosis program. We provide a brief description of the activities that precede BRAC's first pilot of TB control in 1984 to lay the groundwork. BRAC conducted two phases of pilot programs over ten years before it was confident that it had developed a community-based model that could be replicated nationally. We dedicate one chapter to describing this experience and the iterations that occurred. National expansion required a shift of mindset towards partnership and scaling up. Chapter 4 takes the readers through the establishment of a partnership agreement with the government in 1994 and the consequential scale of TB control to the national level, catalyzed by the infusion of resources from the Global Fund in 2004. The choreography of coordinating a multiple stakeholder strategy is complex; in Chapter 5, we focus on the activities and organization of the public-private partnership for TB control in Bangladesh.

In Chapter 6, we examine the community health worker model in depth, with particular attention to how it "fits" and the supervision mechanisms it includes. Chapters 7 and 8 recognize that a delivery model's effectiveness in one context is no guarantee that it can be replicated elsewhere and explore BRAC's work in TB control in Bangladesh's rapidly growing urban areas and rural Afghanistan. Having described all the activities on the ground, in Chapter 9 we move up to the executive office and describe high-level operations and management that enables smooth and sustained delivery on the frontlines. We discuss in Chapter 10 how this model might be applied to other pressing health challenges, such as HIV/AIDS and non-communicable diseases, and finally offer in Chapter 11 a few conclusions we've distilled from this body of experience.

1.2 Peeling the organizational onion

"Everything should be made as simple as possible, but no simpler."

Albert Einstein

The book is written with a broad audience in mind. We've tried to avoid delving too deeply into the technical details or relying on the myriad acronyms of the global health discourse to keep the focus on a system-level analysis and reflection. The delivery of health goods and services, especially in large-scale programs, is inherently complex, and while it is tempting to try to cull a neat list of best practices or lessons learned, we attempt here to represent the complexity itself, without simplifications, and hope to create the opportunity for readers to take away a more comprehensive picture of BRAC. We have assumed a basic familiarity with TB control strategies and concepts, but those desiring more background information on these topics should refer to Appendix A for a brief discussion. TB control is just one small program within BRAC: we've included several exhibits for reference in Appendix B to provide a more comprehensive snapshot of the organization.

Despite the emphasis on a systemic perspective, readers will find quotations and stories woven through the book. BRAC has a strong institutional identity, which has been part in part by the years of commitment and dedication of countless individuals. Many of BRAC's senior leaders grew up with the program, starting as field staff and moving up the ranks as they gained experience and BRAC needed leaders to nurture new initiatives. These stories offer a deeper glimpse at a few of the threads that come together to create the BRAC fabric.

We have identified past failures and current challenges in this book to provide readers with an honest perspective on the program. Leaders working in development are faced with tough decisions every day—the resources will never be sufficient to immediately address all the world's problems. Tradeoffs are a constant element of all operations that good programs must strategically confront. Do we wait for more data or do we implement now? Should we focus on making existing services better or expanding the catchment area? Is a problem local or indicative of a need to change the overall model? Are field staff ready for the decentralization of decision-making on this program or is central supervision still necessary? How do we create systems and processes that can adapt and respond allow programs to work effectively within their means? We have no illusions that BRAC is always on the mark, but the systems BRAC has developed illustrate one example of how an organization can enable rapid identification of weaknesses and motivate constant improvement.

1.3 Background on Bangladesh

Few countries have undergone as much change in the past forty years as Bangladesh. Emerging in 1971 from a bloody fight for liberation from Pakistan, it was termed by former U.S. Secretary of State, Henry Kissinger as "the world's basket case." With forty years of hindsight, how wrong he was. Bangladesh's economy is steadily growing at a rate of 5% per year (Gapminder, 2008). From a health perspective, what it's achieved has literally been referred to by some experts as "a miracle" (Gapminder, 2011). Life expectancy has increased from 44 to 62 since independence, and child mortality has fallen from a staggering rate of 25% to 7%. Fertility rates, which at independence were close to 7, now average 2.9. The declines in the maternal mortality ratio, 1,329 per 100,000 in 1971 to 194 in 2010, also speak to the level of change that Bangladesh has undergone (Gapminder, 2011; National Institute of Population Research and Training et al., 2010). Underlying many of these changes has been the remarkable increase in women's literacy from under 20% in 1980 to rates over 50% (UNESCO, 2007; BBS, 2011).

Average income is currently US $1,883 (purchasing power parity), though half the population lives on under US $1.25 a day

(Gapminder, 2011; Klugman, 2010). A third of the country now resides in urban areas (World development indicators database, 2009). These migrating populations include a sizeable number of young, single women seeking employment in the growing garment industry. Gender norms and social dynamics are shifting in several dimensions. Access to media, information, and communication creates higher levels of international exposure among the younger generation in particular. Subscriptions to mobile phones are growing, jumping from 11% to 64% in the past five years (BBS, 2011).

Yet the challenges remain great. The changes have also resulted in new forms of inequality and next-generation health and social issues. Bangladesh's health infrastructure faces huge challenges in human resources; there are just three doctors for every 10,000 people, and a growing burden of chronic diseases promises to create new strains (WHO, 2007). Community-based programs and public health campaigns are crucial to address these gaps in service delivery. But as only 57% of Bangladeshis are literate, creative strategies are needed for mobilization and awareness raising (BBS, 2011).

Climate change threatens the already flood-prone country, which has experienced two significant cyclones in the past five years. The United Nations Development Program estimates that 10% of Bangladesh's population is affected by natural disasters annually, and this proportion is only expected to increase (Klugman, 2010). If sea levels rise, many of Bangladesh's fertile areas will no longer be arable, compromising its ability to feed its population. Rising food prices worldwide and the related political uprisings internationally underscore the centrality these issues have in determining Bangladesh's future. Today's challenges may look and feel different than those facing BRAC in the 1970s, but they are formidable. BRAC has recognized the need to evolve its strategies to reflect the changing landscape.

Reflection on past actions is critical to future success. We invite the reader to join us in thoughtful exploration of BRAC's TB program to take stock of the organization's achievements to date and how to best prepare for the challenges that the future holds.

Chapter 2

BRAC's Beginnings: Early Experiments in Health

2.1 BRAC's early origins

BRAC was founded by Sir Fazle Hasan Abed, a Bangladeshi trained as a charter accountant who returned from England in 1969 to work for Shell Oil Company in Chittagong.[1] Following the cyclone that occurred in November 1970, he felt compelled by the suffering and devastation he observed to join the relief efforts, becoming the member of HELP, a local, hastily formed organization working in the deeply affected island of Manpura. During the Liberation War in 1971, Abed returned to England to mobilize political support for the creation of Bangladesh and within a few months went to India to work with refugees. Upon returning to his home country after the war ended in December, he decided to found his own non-profit relief organization. He named it the Bangladesh Rehabilitation Assistance Committee (BRAC). It focused on serving 200 villages in Sulla and nearby sub-districts, as he felt that nationwide relief efforts would not reach this area due to its remoteness. BRAC's initial activities included building houses, rehabilitating agriculture and distributing fishing nets and boats to fishermen.

Abed initially assumed that an organization like BRAC would only be necessary for a few years before the government would take over these types of activities. Once the relief and rehabilitation phase was over, he realized the immensity of the challenges and changed his mind. In 1973, BRAC's name was changed to "Bangladesh Rural Advancement Committee" in order to better suit its longer-term mission.[2] BRAC

---

[1] Smillie writes extensively about Sir Fazle Hasan Abed in his recent book *Freedom from Want.*

[2] Over the years, BRAC has ceased to be an acronym and the organization's formal name is now simply "BRAC."

expanded to Manikganj, a sub-district near Dhaka. "When BRAC was started in 1972, we thought that it would probably be needed for two to three years, by which time the national government would consolidate and take control of the situation...[but] after 16 years, we feel that we have not yet outlived our utility and need to do more and more (Abed in Chowdhury and Cash, 1996, 39)."

From BRAC's inception, Abed engaged communities in program planning and constantly evaluated BRAC's efforts. While producing only mixed results at best, early programs exposed BRAC to the complexity and magnitude of village power dynamics. He and his colleagues realized that if they truly wanted to help the poor, they could not continue to conduct activities at the village level, nor consider the "marginalized" as one cohesive population, as villagers themselves tended to group themselves differently.[3] In 1975, BRAC moved from a "whole village" to a "target group" approach in response to these improved understandings. Initial target groups were landless, fishermen, and women, with a focus on serving the poorer sections of each.

Like many other organizations at that time, BRAC saw group formation as an important part of consciousness building and empowerment. It brought individuals together in village organizations to create a collective body. There was great disagreement within BRAC about what its objectives and group activities should include. One question was whether BRAC should provide credit and economic programs to village groups (Smillie 1997, 23). Some vehemently argued that BRAC should focus solely on building the consciousness and advocacy skills that would empower the poor to successfully demand access to public services and resources. These were central questions to BRAC's identity and emerging philosophy. For many years, BRAC would run two models in parallel to observe the results: some groups had both consciousness-raising and economic programs, and others just the former. BRAC found that where it was teaching villagers hard skills and providing access to capital, better results were seen, and this began to form the basis of BRAC's core development strategy.

BRAC was explicit in its "learning by doing" philosophy, often acknowledging the limitations of its certainty in communication with

---

[3] Martha Chen's book, *A silent revolution,* catalogs her observations and analysis from her time in rural villages of Bangladesh in the 1980s.

donors. For example, one 1975 project proposal stated "… as yet we don't know whether to retain the lady family planning organizer as a 'people's healer' or whether to keep the roles separate(Smillie, 2009)." In fact, the position was found to be ineffective and was eliminated. By demonstrating an iterative process that led to better results, BRAC was able to engage donors in its learning process and gain their support for an evolving approach.

> "Some people, in trying to admire village folk, proclaim glibly that the farmer knows best. BRAC does not go along with this. More often than not, it is precisely because of a lack of knowledge of what is best, that the farmer is exploited. If knowledge is power, then ignorance is lack of power, and powerlessness is an attraction for exploitation. The biggest exploiter of the poor is their own ignorance, and though sometimes aware of it, a poor farmer has no way of removing it."
>
> *BRAC Project Proposal, 1975 (Smillie 1997, 15)*

Many of BRAC's early internal memos also indicate that its leadership wanted to distinguish its approach from the other development organizations that had cropped up in Bangladesh following independence. In particular, how to crystallize its conception of empowerment and constructively engage communities were areas of deep exploration.

Many of BRAC's future programs would embody this sentiment—BRAC would discuss needs and approaches at length with the community, but simultaneously incorporate its own wisdom and expert input into the decision-making process. In addition, BRAC was becoming increasingly aware of the structural elements of power and marginalization. Its descriptions reflect sensitivity to these themes in designing programs, and it sought to tackle these fundamental issues as well as their more proximate consequences.

By 1979, BRAC had established a rural credit and training project in three sub-districts. The product of many experiments, the project's activities now included: group formation for the poorest of the poor (with separate groups for men and women), provision of collateral-free credit for income-generating activities, and promotion of agricultural technologies, such as deep tubewells for irrigation, silk production, and poultry rearing.

Organizing poor women into "village organizations" would prove to be a crucial activity for many of BRAC's subsequent activities.

Village organizations provided women with access to group-based microfinance, training on basic accounting, and an opportunity to create a sense of community. Informally, the weekly group meetings provided a forum to discuss local issues, problem solve, and offer support to one another. As BRAC staff sat in these meetings, it heard women discuss health problems they faced: children lost, debt accumulated when a relative's illness required treatment, lack of income when a husband fell ill. To seriously attack poverty, BRAC would need to think about how to address health challenges at the community level.

2.2 Early experiments in health

In 1972, BRAC established four clinics staffed by medical doctors in Sulla. It started training paramedics in 1973. After receiving 12 months of training, paramedics began to carry out vaccination campaigns, work on village sanitation programs, and incorporate public health education in adult education programs (Smillie, 1997, 15). Villagers paid a small fee for service and were treated for minor illnesses. The clinics had the capacity to test and treat TB, though patients were not directly observed while taking treatment. BRAC also trained community health volunteers, popularly known as *shasthya sheboks* and *shasthya shebikas* (male and female health volunteers, respectively), to diagnose ten common conditions and assist the paramedics.

All local health workers were volunteers for BRAC. Without a salary, these individuals depended on the community's willingness to purchase their services for an income. BRAC believed that this was more sustainable than a salary and created a sense of local accountability. However, BRAC noted that many villagers seemed unable or unwilling to pay for services when they needed them.

Beginning in 1974, BRAC encouraged villagers to purchase a health insurance scheme. For a price of five kilograms of unhusked rice at the time of harvest, a household received a year's worth of coverage. While the project was able to recuperate about 30% of its costs through this scheme, BRAC found that it was largely the richer segment of the community that benefited, not BRAC's target groups. Additionally, there were significant variations in quality and behavior at the paramedic level, and BRAC found it difficult to monitor their activities and prevent them from serving as village doctors. This program was discontinued in 1975.

As the government expanded its health system, the need for BRAC's fixed sites diminished. It could be more effective now in linking patients to the government facilities than providing direct treatment. In addition, the *sheboks* and *shebikas* were proving quite effective at treating basic health conditions and BRAC concluded that paramedics at the village level had limited added benefit. It began to plan for a scaled-up pilot of *sheboks* and *shebikas* in Manikganj.

These new experiments gave BRAC new insights into how to design effective programs. It observed that true participation led to low dropout rates, giving it a quick measure of how well its programs fostered engagement. Field-level supervision was crucial for maintaining service delivery projects. Understanding the impact of programs required more than monitoring simple metrics of overall utilization; BRAC's health programs were often primarily serving the village elite. These initiatives were successful in the sense that they had impact, but ultimately failed to fulfill BRAC's objective of benefiting the poor. Without deeper investigation, these differences could go unnoticed. Thorough monitoring would be central to determining which programs should be sustained and scaled.

BRAC was shaped and nurtured by Abed's thoughtful management. Cultivating leadership in others was central to his style, and he was known by his colleagues for his great ability to lead by listening, motivating and inspiring. One observer writes, "If anything BRAC's evolution has mirrored the personality of its founder. A strong desire to do things well engendered the learning culture. His early background in the private sector gave him a keen sense of accounting, accountability and order. His own confidence inspired confidence in others, and 'confidence' has now become almost synonymous with 'empowerment' (Smillie, 1997, 31)."

Far from distancing himself from the village people, Abed had an open-door policy to community members and often engaged in informal discussions with them. Frustration at systematic exploitation that they observed was a frequent motivation for the visits. "'Members are being cheated by the elite because they can't read!' They would complain, and Abed would encourage an active response, 'then start a literacy program' (Nobukatsu Ishikawa, pers comm)." Given the political context and history, most villages lacked access to basic public infrastructure—schools and hospitals were limited in number. When one became ill, private and often unqualified practitioners in the village were the most popular source of care. These doctors frequently doubled as moneylenders, so patients who could not afford treatment would find themselves in great financial debt upon recovery. Village organization leaders raised this issue with Abed, who began to envision ways to help the community gain ownership over its health.

2.3 Research and evaluation

BRAC's Research and Evaluation Division (RED) was established in 1975 when Mushtaque Chowdhury joined the team. RED was BRAC's "eyes and ears" and conducted independent investigations and evaluations. All implementing programs were required to have a built-in budget to support RED's activities. At the end of each year, program and RED staff met to determine the research questions and areas for assessment for the coming year. Some of the early research topics in health included: use patterns of oral contraceptive in rural Bangladesh (1978), an evaluation of BRAC's program on health care (1978), and an assessment of diarrheal interventions in rural Bangladesh (1980). RED was a critical resource in for evaluating programs and determining whether each should be expanded or discontinued.

2.4 *Shasthya shebikas* and *sheboks*: Community health volunteers

In preparation for training community volunteers in Manikganj, BRAC compiled a set of curative and preventative goods that lay people could distribute safely and found that the resulting basket addressed almost 80% of the disease burden in an average village. It then sought the input of the village organizations asking, "Who should be the health agent in your village?" The job did not require extensive training, but it did require community trust and legitimacy. Village organization members, embedded in their community, clearly understood the local social dynamics better than BRAC staff. They nominated

---

Conditions addressed by the *shasthya shebikas* and *sheboks*

1. Anemia
2. Fever
3. Angular stomatitis
4. Iodine deficiency (goiter)
5. Peptic ulcer disease
6. Pneumonia
7. Diarrhea
8. Dysentery
9. Worm infestation
10. Skin disease (scabies, eczema)

members from the group to serve as community health volunteers. *Sheboks* and *shebikas* received six weeks of training from paramedics, who were transferred from Sulla, and were provided the medications at cost (Rohde, 2005, 27). BRAC wanted volunteers to be invested in their work and therefore asked them to purchase the medications, which would be sold at up to a 10% markup. As most of the volunteers were illiterate, one of BRAC's staff from Sulla, Monoronjan Sarkar, created a color-based labeling system for the medications so that they could identify them. Volunteers were instructed to refer complex cases to paramedics or public sector facilities. Between 1977 and 1983, 168 community health volunteers were trained (Islam, Chowdhury, Sarker, 1991).

Within a few years, BRAC observed that *shebikas* were outperforming their male counterparts (*sheboks*). *Shebikas* were informally creating opportunities to discuss health issues in their villages and worked more closely with the paramedics. In addition, *sheboks* had limited access to women and children and appeared to be more motivated to sell goods than to improve health. BRAC was increasingly focusing its microfinance efforts on women as well, and as the village organizations became exclusively female, so too did BRAC's workforce of community health volunteers.

> I have been working as a *shasthya shebika* for a long time, since 1977. Women were not allowed to go out at that time. They also were not allowed to go to the hospital in Manikganj. The people said that NGOs will convert your religion. I decided that I would work for the country and serve the people of the country. I will make them aware and teach them. At that time, very few women worked outside. I was involved to make them aware. I taught them by my own hand. I used to walk a long way to teach them on how to make home-made rehydration saline.
>
> *Pariskrunnesa, shasthya shebika in Muljan, Manikganj*
> *(Ishikawa, unpublished)*

2.5 Learning the scale: The oral therapy extension program

Many of BRAC's initial experiments in health focused on impact and sustainability, not on scalability. Its decision to launch a large program to take on one of the leading killers of children marked the beginning of scale as one of BRAC's priorities for its programs. It would also prove to be instructive in helping BRAC codify a process of scaling up.

In 1970, the childhood mortality rate in Bangladesh (East Pakistan) was 250 per 1,000, with diarrheal disease as a leading cause

(Gapminder, 2011; Chowdhury and Cash, 1996, 21). Researchers in East Pakistan demonstrated the effectiveness of oral rehydration therapy in facility and community settings. During Bangladesh's war for independence, doctors working in refugee camps in West Bengal, India demonstrated the effectiveness of oral rehydration in managing diarrhea during cholera outbreaks in this displaced population. They relied heavily on the efforts of lay people, such as family members, to monitor patients and administer the therapy, and achieved a mortality rate of under 5% (Chowdhury and Cash, 1996, 21). BRAC saw an opportunity to democratize the knowledge still further, reckoning that the average mother could be taught to prepare the solution at home, using the common household ingredients of salt, *gur* (unrefined brown sugar), and water.[4] However, the World Health Organization (WHO) recommended against home-made solutions, encouraging BRAC instead to share information and generate demand for pre-made packets of ORT and facility-based care. After conducting its own feasibility studies, BRAC decided to proceed with its initial plan for the Oral Therapy Extension Program (OTEP). Its research demonstrated that mothers could reliably produce the solution, and given the huge barriers to accessing care and the limited supply of oral rehydration therapy in Bangladesh at the time, the strategy of empowering families to treat diarrhea at home offered the most potential for impact. This decision was strongly condemned at the time by experts at the WHO because they wanted a program where ORT packets were the only option. A few even approached the government of Bangladesh and BRAC's donors to try to obstruct OTEP's implementation. Nevertheless, the government approved BRAC's plans, and it forged ahead.

BRAC trained hundreds of health workers to conduct home visits and educational activities for the community. Using pay-for-performance incentives with carefully designed monitoring and evaluation activities, BRAC was able to ensure quality and reward real-time innovations in the field. In its ten-year lifespan, OTEP reached nearly 12 million mothers across Bangladesh, contributing to the precipitous drop in child mortality that Bangladesh enjoyed in its post-independence era (Chowdhury and Cash, 1996). Evaluation studies comparing death rates before and after OTEP found that post

---

[4] This description is quite brief. Readers interested in the operational details and epidemiological results of the project should see Chowdhury and Cash's *A Simple Solution*.

natal deaths dropped by 14% (71 to 61 per 1,000 live births) and childhood deaths dropped 37% (27 to 17 per 1,000 children age 1-4) (Chowdhury and Cash, 1996, 99).

In reflecting on the campaign, senior leaders felt that they had learned several valuable lessons that could be applied to future health programs. These included:

1. Using data allowed them to make improvements quickly. Evaluation was a continuous process.

2. When motivated, field workers were adept at making small improvements that could greatly improve results. Tying their compensation to mother's retention of information and ability to prepare the solution led to many small-scale refinements on the front lines.

3. Pay-for-performance requires a supervision system with the capacity to accurately assess performance. Only with these supports would the incentives produce the desired results.

4. Lay persons can effectively provide basic health services at the community level.

In addition, the experience of taking a program to scale was one that significantly affected the thinking of BRAC's leaders. Scaling up a program to the size achieved by OTEP proved to be "a whole different ball game" from managing a smaller-scale project (Mushtaque Chowdhury, pers comm). One serious challenge in maintaining quality at scale proved to be mid-level staff. BRAC's own reports cautioned against expanding too rapidly, pointing to the lower levels of information retention observed in mothers

> "Do we serve our people as best we can out of the kind of poverty, the intense dire poverty, that we have in our country? Do we remain small and beautiful or do we scale up and try to take the consequences. BRAC has decided to try to take the consequences of becoming large."
>
> Sir Fazle Hasan Abed, BRAC (Smillie 2009)

trained during these shortages relative to mothers trained in other years (Chowdhury and Cash, 1996, 104).

2.6 Conclusions

Many of BRAC's initial leaders did not have a formal background in development work. The organization's early years were characterized by experimentation, supported by developing mechanisms for data collection and analysis. Simultaneously, an organizational culture that embraced innovation and constant improvement began to germinate. These characteristics would prove to be fundamental to BRAC's long-term development and identity. These years were also formative in BRAC's approach to development. Starting with fairly simple activities of providing income-generating materials, it added consciousness building, skills building, group formation, health services, new technologies, and education. The cumulative effect was a presence in the community that served as a platform for new programs and initiatives. Simultaneously, BRAC's health activities increasingly centered on female community health volunteers. As *shebikas* demonstrated competence in providing basic health education and products, BRAC began to consider what other activities they were capable of performing. In this regard, they were often ahead of the international experts.

The OTEP experience was a watershed moment because it established a framework for scaling up and demonstrated the potential impact of lay health workers. The OTEP experience also affected BRAC on a more abstract level. Its leaders were not aware of any national programs completely administered by NGOs. OTEP demonstrated that BRAC had the potential to think at the national scale and gave them the courage to take subsequent programs to scale more readily. In looking through internal and external publications at the time, one can observe the increasing enthusiasm of moving towards scale.

BRAC was also struck by the loyalty that several individuals in its donor organizations had to the program, refusing to cede their support in the face of significant pressure from expert bodies. In particular, the Swiss Development Cooperation and the Swedish Free Church Aid. provided the crucial funding to kick start the scale up efforts.[5]

BRAC's leadership noted the power in demonstrating the possibility of an idea. Despite its initial resistance, once BRAC empirically demonstrated success in OTEP, previous critics, such as UNICEF, began to provide support to the program. Through

---

[5] Support from the Swedish International Development Agency would replace support from the Swedish Free Church Aid during the life of the project.

engagement with the international community and dissemination of its successes, BRAC could ensure that others benefited from its discoveries. This would prove an important lesson for TB control, another area in which BRAC chose to push the international community to embrace a community-based model for treatment.

Chapter 3

Piloting a Community-based Tuberculosis Program

"It took 10 years of piloting community-based TB control before we scaled. But that's how long it took for us to gain the confidence to grow."

Faruque Ahmed, BRAC

3.1 Assessing program feasibility

BRAC's *shasthya shebika* (health volunteer) was one of many lay health worker models arising during the 1970s, as the concept gained popularity in many developing countries searching for strategies to better reach underserved rural communities that lacked access to formal medical settings. BRAC's *shebika* program did not supplant the need for a functioning health system, but it created access to basic goods, information and referrals. In most cases, the *shebika's* range of responsibilities was restricted to preventative goods, such as iron pills, or treatment for acute conditions, such as oral rehydration therapy for diarrhea. These conditions could be identified easily and had straightforward regimens with limited side effects.

When the *shebikas* identified tuberculosis (TB) as a major health problem in their communities and asked BRAC to help them address it, the prospect of *shebikas* administering treatment posed more complexities to consider. At the time, tuberculosis required twelve months of daily treatment, including injections several times a week during the first two months. Failure to complete treatment could lead to acquisition of drug resistance. TB treatment in Bangladesh was only administered in the 44 chest clinics, 8 TB segregation hospitals and 6 specialty hospitals. BRAC's leadership was unaware of any programs attempting to treat tuberculosis with lay persons in a community setting, in Bangladesh or elsewhere.

And yet, it was clear that tuberculosis fit squarely within BRAC's mission. National prevalence was 870 per 100,000 population, and the majority of TB cases occurred in those ages 15-59, on whom family income depended (Chowdhury et al., 1991). Without treatment, TB led to death. The rural poor were unlikely to access the government sites, which required transport to and from the facilities and steep costs for the long medical treatment. Adherence support was not provided to patients, and treatment completion rates were around 25% (Chowdhury et al., 1992). From all angles, it was evident that the need was great. But could BRAC take this on? Could TB be addressed in a community setting by lay health workers?

Simultaneously, there was interest from the government of Bangladesh in gaining a better understanding of the prevalence of tuberculosis. In 1983, Japanese physician Yuichi Koseki conducted a prevalence survey under the guidance of the National TB Program in Manikganj. BRAC and the National Anti-Tuberculosis Association of Bangladesh (NATAB) both provided technical support and human resources for the research. Participating in the study gave BRAC the momentum to pilot a TB program.

3.2 Pilot: Phase one

BRAC decided to test community-based TB treatment in Manikganj to see if the *shebikas* could provide effective supervision. A team was formed to run the pilot program and consisted of BRAC and NATAB staff, with significant guidance from Nobukatsu Ishikawa, a physician from Japan's Research Institute of Tuberculosis who specialized in community programming. He received funding from Japanese Overseas Christian Services to assist with program design and implementation. BRAC's team included Aminul Alam, Jalaluddin Ahmed, Mushtaque Chowdhury and Nazrul Islam. Other institutions also participated significantly; NATAB's Secretary General Sakhawat Hussain and his junior colleague Akramul Islam helped manage the pilot and the National Tuberculosis Program's (NTP) Md. Shirajul Islam, Khurshid Alam Hyder, Gulam Nabi, Dilrose Banu, Jalal Uddin Ahmed and Vikarunnessa Begum participated regularly. BRAC's programs in Manikganj at the time covered about 235 villages, with a total population of 220,000. In the pilot, 168 *shebikas* were trained in TB activities (Islam, Chowdhury, Sarker, 1991). *Shebikas* went door-to-door in their communities, inquiring whether any residents have suffered from a cough for more than four weeks. When an individual answered affirmatively, the *shebika* would instruct the individual on how to produce a morning sputum sample. She would accompany the patient (unless the patient was too sick to travel) to mobile sputum collection and smearing sites that branch offices held regularly where the program organizer took two sputum samples per patient for testing at the laboratory that BRAC established in the Manikganj office. The NTP provided training to a BRAC staff member who would perform the sputum smear test. After confirmation by a medical officer, the diagnosis would be communicated to the patient by the *shebika*. She also oversaw the 12-month treatment regimen and provided the injections during the intensive phase (details in Figure 3.1). All treatment was provided in the village, except in cases of side effects, which were referred to government facilities.

Ishikawa was aware that one of the greatest challenges the program would face was that of adherence: treatment at that time required a year's worth of daily oral medications and injections every other day for the first two months. To gain insights on how others had tackled the issue of adherence, Ishikawa visited other health programs in Bangladesh and found a French NGO in the Shariakandi *upazila* (sub-district) of Bogra, Brothers to All Men, providing services to the poor that required its patients to put down a bond for TB treatment that was returned at the conclusion of the treatment. Defaulters forfeited the bond. Ishikawa thought that this modification could improve the adherence for BRAC's patients as well. Patients were asked to deposit Tk 100 (US $3), about a week's worth of wages, before treatment was initiated. At the completion of treatment (including the collection of sputum), Tk 75 was returned to them, and Tk 25 given to the attending *shebika* for her provision of treatment support activities (Chowdhury et al., 1991). Patients and BRAC signed a contract before initiating treatment that outlined these terms. BRAC considered only paying *shebikas* for successful completion in keeping with its incentive philosophy, but this proved operationally difficult when patients dropped out mid-treatment for no particular reason, migrated out, discontinued treatment due to side effects, or died. In practice, *shebikas* were compensated for their support except in cases where treatment was discontinued in the intensive phase. When a patient lacked the funds to produce the bond, BRAC asked the village organization to post a bond for them, or would waive the bond entirely. No one was denied treatment if they tested positive for TB.

Figure 3.1: Details on diagnosis protocol and treatment regimen, 1984-1994

Treatment component	Protocol
Regimen for intensive phase (2 months)	30 streptomycin injections, given on alternate days; isoniazid and thiacetazone daily
Regimen for continuation phase (10 months)	Isoniazid and thiacetazone daily
Sputum testing during treatment	Testing at end of months 1, 3, 6, 9, 12 during treatment, and 1 month after treatment completion
Protocol for complications	Refer to specialist clinics or hospitals

Reactions from the community

Bengali society at this time was fairly conservative with respect to gender roles. Women were expected to manage household activities and childcare (Afsana et al., 1998). Though many also participated in home-based agricultural, poultry, and animal husbandry, virtually no opportunities for women existed in the formal economy. Rates of malnutrition, illiteracy and other measures of development indicated significant gender inequality.

In choosing women to serve as *shasthya shebikas* in the villages, BRAC was challenging the status quo. There were many in the community who criticized BRAC, at times calling it un-Islamic, and threatened the *shebikas* directly (Sharma, 2002).

> Our village organization initially had seventy members. As the shebika, I faced many pressures from outside. I overcame all these. When I started the *Samity* [Village organization], local elites surrounded my home and snatched my attendance register. They said they would break the *Samity*. They also beat my husband.
>
> I took all *Samity* members to the home of the matbor [local elite]. I said to him, "Either you give us right to grow rice or give us work." We did it in reality! Then he said us to continue the *Samity*.

Some of these leaders had also supported me, mainly the educated people. At that time, educated people were very few. Mostly school teachers helped me. But later this changed. These leaders came to me with sick people [with TB]. If there was no change, would they come to me?"

Maksuda, Shasthya shebika in Bethila, Manikganj
(Ishikawa, unpublished)

The village organization proved to be a key source of strength during these challenges. Members supported the *shebikas* and helped advocate for her value to the community.

Husbands also proved to be an important factor in *shebikas'* activities. Many supported their wives' new opportunities to contribute financially to the household. BRAC tried to keep the workload to a level that did not interfere with other responsibilities women typically had at home. *Shebikas* were expected to spend 2-3 hours a day on health-related activities.

Ultimately, TB patients themselves were critical in establishing the legitimacy of *shebikas*. Members of the community witnessed people with a disease known to be lethal return to health, thanks to treatment provided by BRAC via the *shebika*. These patients often began to encourage others in the community with symptoms of TB to seek out the *shebika*. Even vocal naysayers began to send their family members for treatment, though at times secretly to avoid having to publicly reverse their opinion.

3.3 Experimenting with the model

In reviewing the program data in 1988, BRAC found that the program had identified and treated 187 patients and achieved a 66% of completion rate (Chowdhury et al., 1991). Given the estimates for the prevalence of TB in the area, BRAC felt that case detection rates could be improved substantially. It decided to pilot an incentive strategy, offering *shebikas* Tk 50 (US $1.50) for every new or relapsed case that they identified in their community that tested sputum smear positive. In 1989, *shebikas* initiated 77 patients on treatment. Despite increasing the number of cases detected, this incentive was never scaled. "It worked," Akramul reflected later, "the case detection rate went up. But it was difficult from a management perspective to monitor and confirm that the cases weren't being manipulated."[1] Instead, BRAC increased the bond to Tk 200 and increased the

---

[1] Unless otherwise specified, all quotations are from author interviews and personal correspondence in 2011.

portion retained by the *shebika* to Tk 100, hoping that this would motivate them to find patients and ensure patient adherence to treatment (Chowdhury et al., 1997).

The bond, while financial in nature, represented a new innovation on BRAC's part. Without moving to a fee-for-service model, BRAC had found a way to engage patients in an active transaction for their health care. Patients were recognized as partners and decision makers in their care. In addition, the process of signing the bond agreement emphasized the contract between BRAC and the patient in an active manner.

On a broader level, the TB program represented a significant expansion of the role of the *shebika*. BRAC was now tasking them with active case finding throughout the village, which conflicted with some of the prevailing norms limiting women's social behaviors. The consequences for *shebikas* and their families were at times quite severe, requiring BRAC to confront whether it could justify its strategy.

> "In Bangladesh, cash is scarce and always kept by men. The same is true for power. When BRAC's programs started giving women access to loans and other new things, it created an imbalance in the family with respect to power. Women were gaining power, and it was difficult for men to accept it. This can lead to violence. But over time, a man sees how the woman manages the money. She spends it on the family, her children's education; it's not being wasted on tobacco and so on. He also sees that there is a huge organization like BRAC supporting this woman, and he can't just ignore it or defeat it. That's how social change happens, and how an intervention can have an impact on an individual's life."
>
> *Mushtaque Chowdhury, Rockefeller Foundation, formerly BRAC*

While the program's explicit focus was TB, its approach embodied larger goals of social change. It would take longer to change norms than to treat a few cases of TB, but the visible proof of the *shebika*'s ability to cure patients of what was widely considered a fatal illness was a powerful change agent. Despite initial social conflict, BRAC could observe that given time, the *shebika* could gain legitimacy and support for her work.

During these years, Ishikawa simultaneously conducted a study to rigorously evaluate community-based health volunteers, comparing areas with no community component, areas with a community group (though not health specific), and areas where groups included a community health volunteer. Villages with groups were more likely to be aware of preventive public health information (use of latrines, etc.), and those groups with a volunteer were more likely to think that health issues could be tackled at the village level. Compared to other villagers, group members were more likely to change health behaviors, such as adopting family planning or ensuring their children were vaccinated (Ishikawa, 1992). With these findings, BRAC had compelling evidence for its village organization and *shebika* approach to TB and other public health programs.

3.4 International exposure

Like the other members of the team working in Manikganj, Mushtaque was keenly aware that any successes BRAC had in these experiments could be hugely informative for TB control efforts in low-income countries around the world. In 1989, Arata Kochi, WHO, invited him to a small conference in Boston to present the program's results to date. "The interest of that audience, all of whom were experts in TB at the time, was really encouraging, and only confirmed the fact that we had to be sure to document and disseminate our results broadly," said Mushtaque.

A full description of the program results was published in the newsletter of the International Union Against TB and Lung Disease (Chowdhury et al., 1991). In addition, the team wrote a letter to the *Lancet* sharing the key details: BRAC's pilot from 1984-1989 had overall treated 264 cases with a completion rate of 60% and an average cost of US $108 per case. The authors concluded, "The BRAC program has demystified the treatment of TB in Bangladesh and the committee plans to expand coverage to 2 million or so by the end of 1993 (Chowdhury et al., 1992)."

Others within Bangladesh were paying attention to these early pilots as well. Khurshid Alam Hyder, WHO, commented, "As early as 1985 I went to see BRAC's project in Manikganj. It was pretty impressive to see how strongly the *shebika* got behind the patient. The model looked promising, even at that time."

Armed with internal consensus and outside approbation, BRAC decided to pursue opportunities to scale up the TB program. The first step would be to create the capacity within BRAC for this endeavor by creating a position on its staff for a TB program manager. Mushtaque asked Akramul, NATAB, if he'd be interested in overseeing the effort. Already planning to pursue a master's in public health, Akramul accepted the offer informally and planned to join once he completed his studies.

3.5 Tightening the *shebika* model

In 1991, RED did an in-depth analysis of the *shebika* program in Manikganj to investigate variation in individual performance and assess the model's feasibility to be scaled to ten sub-districts. *Shebikas* were predominantly married women in their thirties with less than two years of schooling (Islam, Chowdhury, Sarker, 1991). All were members of their local village organization. Characteristics associated with relatively high performance were gender (female outperformed males), basic literacy, and currently being married. Higher performers also spent about twice as much time on *shebika* activities as others, averaging 22 hours a week compared with 12 for low-performers (Islam, Chowdhury, Sarker, 1991). Monthly income averaged Tk 137 (US $1.96).[2]

About 16% of the entire cohort had dropped out, on average after four years of active service, citing a variety of reasons including family programs and husbands' disapproval. High performing *shebikas* (i.e. those who generated more income) were much less likely to drop out (Islam, Chowdhury, Sarker, 1991). Many participated for income generation, but social work was the predominant reason mentioned in interviews (Islam, Chowdhury, Sarker, 1991). *Shebikas* appeared to take advantage of many of BRAC's programs simultaneously, with significant proportions participating in trainings on poultry rearing and traditional birth attendant activities (Islam, Chowdhury, Sarker, 1991).

Program organizers often were completely unfamiliar with *shebika* activities and responsibilities, indicating weaknesses in the supervision system (Islam, Chowdhury, Sarker, 1991). Patient registries were not regularly maintained by the *shebikas*, nor checked by their supervisors. When tested on their knowledge and prescribing habits,

---

[2] For an "upgraded" *shebika*, which resembles the current model. At one point BRAC also had a less trained cadre that was discontinued. Their average monthly income was Tk 55.

researchers found that *shebikas* generally were well informed and had sound practices. But few formal mechanisms existed to regulate their activities. In theory, the village organization could provide a measure of accountability, as the *shebikas'* main clientele were its members and their children (Islam, Chowdhury, Sarker, 1991).

When questioned about what they would do if BRAC withdrew the program, the vast majority of *shebikas* opined that they would simply buy the medications from the market and continue to conduct similar activities (Islam, Chowdhury, Sarker, 1991). If BRAC ceased to provide training, some indicated that they would advocate for the public sector to support their efforts in this capacity.

3.6 Phase two of the pilot

"We were scaling up a comprehensive health and development program to ten sub-districts, and here we had this TB model that we thought worked and was ready to be scaled up. We decided to integrate it into the program to see how it worked."

Sadia Chowdhury, World Bank, formerly BRAC

BRAC had scaled organically in the 1970s and 1980s, expending more energy on experimentation and gaining a deep understanding of village dynamics. In the late 1980s, aided by the successes of the OTEP program and its promising TB program, it began to focus more aggressively on horizontal expansion. The shifting focus and decision to grow had significant implications for program management.

BRAC's core, *shebika*-based health program was called the essential health care program and was managed jointly with microfinance as the rural development program. Increasingly, these activities were funded through their cost recovery mechanisms and BRAC's revenue from social enterprise ventures. Grants received for other health projects were managed by the health and population division. These included many "programs," but programs were simply the funded projects and usually dissolved once the grant was completed. In many ways, the health and population division functioned as a laboratory for new health experiments. The resources from these grants enabled BRAC to focus intensely on evaluating and refining new models. If an intervention proved to be effective and seemed scalable, it could be integrated into the essential health care program and spread through BRAC's entire catchment area.

In 1991, Sadia Chowdhury took over the health and population division at BRAC, which had just received three-year grants from UNICEF, the Swedish International Development Agency (SIDA), and the United Kingdom's Department for International Development (DFID) to launch a women's health and development program in ten sub-districts. The program aimed to provide comprehensive health services, including pre and post-natal care, sanitized delivery practices, immunization, nutritional care services, and treatment for acute respiratory infections. All services would be delivered by BRAC's *shebikas*. While the primary focus of the grant was on maternal and child health, BRAC saw it as an opportunity to test the feasibility of several promising models for scale. These additions were maternity waiting homes, nutritional support, TB control, treatment for acute respiratory infection, and health centers (*shushasthyas*).

Based on the results of the RED study of *shebika* perform, the central office began to monitor *shebika* selection more closely. The increasing educational attainment of women made finding *shebikas* that had basic literacy skills much more feasible. In addition, the program's funding allowed BRAC to increase the number of field staff, who could provide enhanced support and supervision to the *shebikas*.

In 1993, Akramul formally joined BRAC as the TB program manager and was the only person dedicated to TB programming at the central level. His role was primarily technical: he was to ensure that the program had the information, supplies, training, and support necessary to carry out the program. The medical officers and laboratory technicians that BRAC hired to work at the sub-district level received training from the NTP, which BRAC supplemented with training and support on how to supervision the *shebikas'* activities. BRAC procured its own medications and laboratory consumables and had to manage its own supply chain to the branch offices.

In 1991 and 1992, the women's health and development program's major activity was to select and train new *shebikas* in the villages of the sub-districts that were not already covered. The TB program supervised the establishment of laboratories in BRAC offices. In 1993, they began to enroll patients. During the first two months, *shebikas* visited the patients every other day to provide the injections and oversee treatment. For the final ten months, *shebikas* provided weekly visits to furnish a 7-day supply of medication and adherence support (Afsana et al., 1998).

Given that the delivery model for TB was fairly standardized at this point, the expanded pilot was an opportunity to answer some of the operational questions that would critical if BRAC wanted to scale up. As the program was rolled out across the ten sub-districts, BRAC experimented with different modifications to refine the model. Some of the issues it investigated were the necessary ratio of medical officers on staff and laboratories that BRAC required per sub-district. Another area of interest

> "We'd go and stay for quite a long time, as long as 15 days in some cases. In every sub-district, we'd go, and we'd work just like a program organizer or an area manager. Sitting with the staff for meetings was a regular practice and culture."
>
> *Jalaluddin Ahmed, BRAC*

was where to locate decision making ability—what could be decentralized vs. handled centrally? Akramul reviewed the data regularly to see where there were areas of great variation. The team would follow up with the struggling sites to try to understand whether there were issues in data collection or performance and subsequently provide appropriate support. He also helped the laboratories set up a system of quality assurance (which was not yet required by the NTP) and implement a system of cross-checking 10% of slides between labs. The women's health and development program had a research cell, linked with RED, to provide independent project monitoring and enable BRAC to improve its program more systematically.

BRAC expected its staff to spend significant time in the field, particularly when nurturing new programs. Regional managers were required to spend 15 days a month in the field, and central office staff often spent 15-20 days a month in the field during this time period.

While visiting the programs, staff members maintained a diary. Entries had a specific format and would be signed by supervisors. In addition to reviewing financial and administrative activity, supervisors spoke with the local staff and community health volunteers about how activities were going—what was working, what wasn't. What had they tried recently? Each sub-district had a manager, and they each were implementing distinct innovations. These experiences were recorded and taken back to the headquarters in Dhaka, where staff would share them with directors regularly. Successful innovations would also be disseminated to other sub-districts with the central field staff traveled to other regions.

3.7 Program performance

Many of the activities included in women's health and development program were still in the pilot phase and undergoing experimentation and refinement. The TB program had moved onto the next phase of inquiry, which included questions of impact. Mushtaque oversaw a project at RED that compared TB prevalence in areas with BRAC's TB program to control sub-districts where the government was the provider of care.

In the expanded pilot, *shebikas* identified 3,886 cases of TB in their communities. Ninety percent of patients accepted treatment from BRAC, with the others often preferring to see a physician at a chest clinic or hospital. BRAC believed that some refused based on concerns about confidentiality. Of those that entered BRAC's program, cure rates were 81% (see table). Comparison of the prevalence rate in sub-districts with a BRAC program to a control sub-district found that the prevalence was roughly cut in half by BRAC's program (0.07 vs. 0.15 per 1,000) within four years (Chowdhury et al., 1999).

Table 3.1: BRAC TB program's patient outcomes, 1992-1994

Category	N	%
Number identified as active TB cases	3886	NA
Number of patients accepting treatment	3497	90
Number of patients cured	2431	81
Number of patients completed but not tested at 13 months	402	11
Died during treatment (of any cause)	336	9.6
Failed	51	1.5
Dropped out	109	3.1
AFB negative at 3 months	2972	85
Transferred/migrated/referred	168	4.8

Source: Chowdhury et al., 1999.

BRAC's cure rate had risen substantially during the second phase of the pilot. The acceptance rate was fairly high; the inclusion of the bond as a criterion did not deter most patients. Qualitative research from 1994 indicated that both *shebikas* and patients supported the bond and payment system: they thought that it improved both patient likelihood to adhere and *shebika* motivation to provide support. Willingness and ability to provide the bond was also high; 60% of patients could deposit the bond up front, and most other patients were able to provide a reduced bond or offer the bond in installments (Osaki, 1995). The lost-to-follow-up rate was quite low; BRAC could account for the whereabouts and activity of most of its patients. Most side effects experienced by patients were minor and did not require hospital-based attention. These were very promising indications that the model could be effectively managed at a larger scale.

In addition to yielding relatively successful patient outcomes, another positive indicator of program success was improved community perception of the *shebikas*. RED researchers generally heard high praise from patients and other members of the community. *Shebikas* also reported that they enjoyed their work and did not find it disruptive to their other household responsibilities.

Levels of stigma against TB patients were still significant; half of patients reported isolation from family or negative responses from the community (Chowdhury et al., 1999). BRAC hoped that over time, as the community saw more patients effectively cured, stigma would continue to decline.

3.8 BRAC's evolution as an organization

The transition from a small NGO to one capable of handling a complex portfolio of multi-sectoral programs required new systems and infrastructure. In its health work alone, BRAC was managing approximately 4,500 *shebikas* across Bangladesh (Chowdhury and Chowdhury, 1997). In addition, it was growing at a rate of 2,000 new village organizations annually and planned to increase program coverage by 30% each year for the next decade (Lovell, 1991, 2). Whereas informal collaboration had often led to program breakthroughs in the past, BRAC's size required increasing formalization at the organizational level. Despite its growth, BRAC's greatest value stemmed from its ability to listen at the ground level, and protecting its relationship and responsiveness to community needs would be crucial to maintaining effectiveness.

Human resources

From 1984-1990, BRAC more than doubled the number of full-time staff it employed (see graph below) (Lovell, 1991, 119). Increasingly, BRAC needed to create a formal system to build capacity in its workforce. It also had to ensure that new employees were inculcated with the strong sense of mission that underpinned BRAC's programmatic choices and methodologies. Staff were also expected to acquire a thorough understanding of the communities and appreciation for listening to its ideas and opinions.

BRAC's original team had worked tirelessly to get the organization off the ground. They expected similar levels of commitment from the new members of the team. The hours and expectations were grueling; half of all new program officers resigned in their first year (Lovell, 1991, 119). All program organizers began in a probationary period and spent a year in the field. In addition to the expectations for a strong work ethic, BRAC strove to identify and reward entrepreneurial behavior and experimentation (Lovell, 1991, 119). Feedback was continuous, and field staff received quarterly reports comparing their individual performance to the norm (Lovell, 1991, 149). For those that were committed to BRAC's mission and could handle the pace of work, BRAC could turn into a lifelong employer. Though many quit within the first year, attrition rates overall were below 4% (Smillie, 1997, 25).

Figure 3.2: Full-time BRAC staff, 1983-1990

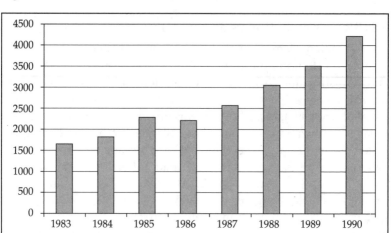

Source: Lovell, 1991.

Stemming from its commitment to local ownership, BRAC's leadership intentionally kept its central office lean and decentralized much decision making (Lovell, 1991, 123). The few individuals charged with providing the overarching leadership were extraordinary as a result, and Abed set up mechanisms to invest in their capabilities over time as well. It was not uncommon for BRAC to encourage and when possible offer financial support to its promising stars to pursue higher education. Mushtaque, who completed a fellowship at Harvard in the early 1990s, and Akramul, who would take time in the late 1990s to pursue his PhD, were just two examples of this policy in practice. Overall, BRAC invested about 7% of its annual budget in staff development. Abed maintained a close touch with the organization—in addition to the open-door policy for staff and members of village organizations, he personally conducted most exit interviews.

BRAC sought strengthen its human resource capacity in anticipation of the challenges that scaling up would provide. In 1990, BRAC launched the management development program, primarily offering short courses for senior level staff and the growing number of mid-level staff, as well as managers from other organizations (Smillie, 1997, 28).

In 1991, Professor Catherine Lovell of the University of California, Los Angeles wrote a book documenting BRAC's characteristics and activities, noting that it was one of the largest non-governmental organizations in the world and winner of several prestigious international awards. She writes of the fluidity of BRAC's operations, "BRAC is large, complex and multifaceted, and because it is continually evolving—learning, adapting, changing, growing—it is difficult at any one moment to capture an accurate picture of the details of all of its activities (Lovell, 1991, 4)."

3.9 External engagement

The public sector

Through its engagement with the government in programs for immunization and TB control, BRAC was gaining appreciation as a partner, particularly in experimentation with new programs. When facing decisions about how to approach nutrition, the government of Bangladesh asked BRAC to pilot a successful program from Tamil Nadu, India to help the government determine if it should adopt the model nationally.

During the Manikganj pilot, BRAC had received medications from the government, though during the expanded pilot, they had used program funds as the national program had reorganized and was focused on its own programmatic expansion. Throughout the pilots, BRAC established its own laboratories in local BRAC offices and used its own staff to conduct the microscopy. There was limited communication with local public sector health officials about its activities.

In 1990, a review by the World Bank found that Bangladesh had a TB case detection rate of under 20% and a cure rate below 50% (Chowdhury and Chowdhury, 1997). With the WHO, the World Bank urged the Ministry of Health and Family Welfare to prioritize the eradication of leprosy and control of TB by the year 2000. A.K. Md. Ahsan Ali, National Institute of Diseases of the Chest and Hospital, was recruited to lead the National TB Program (NTP) in 1991, though with minimal resources. "I remember when they sent someone to visit us from Geneva. We were supposed to be working on a concept paper to present to the Ministry, but we didn't even have a computer. I didn't have a salary, nor did I have money yet to pay my staff. The WHO representative saw that we needed some help and immediately gave us a small grant to give us something to get started with." The concept paper was approved, and in some months, all the staff were officially appointed. During his tenure at the National Institute, Ahsan had practiced clinically and knew that the default rates for TB patients were substantial. "I wanted to publish on the rates, but they were so high, what would I say?" When the WHO approached him about the directly observed therapy, short-course (DOTS) strategy, he was excited at the opportunity to pilot it in Bangladesh (Appendix A includes a description of the DOTS strategy). In 1992-1993, the National TB and Leprosy Control Program focused on implementing DOTS in two sub-districts near Dhaka, Savar and Dhamrai, and then expanded to two more remote sub-districts. Ishikawa and Japan's Research Institute of Tuberculosis provided technical support and research capabilities to the project. Ahsan recalls, "We spent a lot of time in the field trying to understand the challenges. DOTS was so new at the time; everyone was trying to figure out how it would work. We had a lot of visitors from all over the region to come and see how things were working here." Even in these early pilots, the national program began to realize that having NGO involvement would greatly increase the country's capacity for TB control.

Ahsan had no formal involvement in BRAC's programming, but through his relationship with Ishikawa, he received informal reports on their TB program. He was impressed with the infrastructure that they established at the community level and their ability to treat patients in rural areas.

3.10 Financial support

Historically, BRAC had cultivated open and close relationships with donors. Donors often funded the organization, not just discrete project, consistently providing support over many, many grant cycles (Lovell, 1991, 161). In many ways, this allowed BRAC the latitude to experiment. In addition, by 1990, a third of BRAC's resources were self-generated, providing additional independence in its priority setting.

Overall, BRAC's budget increased from Tk 68 million (US $1.3 million) to Tk 2.6 billion (US $47 million), a 40-fold increase over ten years (see graph below). The health budget mirrored this growth, increasing from 17 million (US $0.33 million) to 81 million (US $1.46 million), although in relative terms, health represented a decreasing proportion of BRAC's spending over this time period (25% in 1984 versus 3% in 1994).

Figure 3.3: BRAC's total budget, 1984-1994

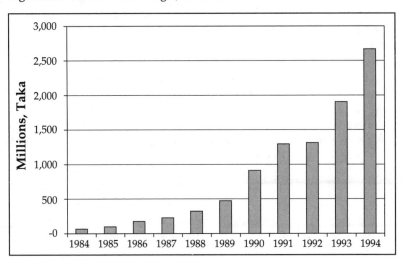

Figure 3.4: BRAC's health budget, 1984-1994

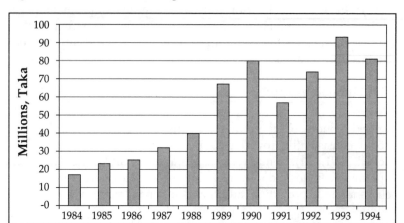

Scaling up programs required scaled up financial resources, including ones that offered a reasonable timeframe. As BRAC grew confident in its delivery models, it began to plan for gaining the necessary commitments to support a major expansion. Past successes would prove to be a significant asset. "When donors signed on for the OTEP expansion, we didn't have a proven track record. They just had to trust us. But, once we demonstrated through that experience that we will be able to identify challenges as they emerged and were prepared to respond, our donors gained a lot of confidence in us as an organization. This really helped when we started to recruit resources to scale up our other programs." Mushtaque explained.

Large-scale programs would require levels of funding that surpassed what many individual donors would be able to give. BRAC needed to find a way to pool resources and commitments from several sources. In 1989, Abed approached BRAC's donors to discuss a collaborative funding effort. BRAC asserted that by creating a consortium, both sides could work more efficiently: BRAC would not need to invest in individual proposals to various donors, and donors could streamline program evaluation by coordinating activities (Lovell, 1991, 157). The Dutch NGO NOVIB, a long-time supporter of BRAC's work, responded positively and was critical in convincing other donors to participate. BRAC presented its plans comprehensively, and with the donors discussed individual commitments within the overall plan.

By 1990, BRAC had a four-year commitment from the consortium for US \$50 million, and a pledge for an additional US \$8.6 million over three years for health programming came in 1991 (Lovell, 1991, 155). Though the women's health and development program received one additional year of funding from DFID, it was clear that the grant would not be renewed. While the other four scaled pilot projects were to be discontinued following the end of the grant, BRAC's health team believed that the TB program should be sustained and scaled. In order to do this, it would need to find support for the significant costs of the medications and lab reagents.

3.11 Conclusions

In developing its model for community-based TB control, BRAC had to test several layers of concepts. The first was whether a *shebika* could provide treatment effectively. In Manikganj, BRAC focused on training and supporting *shebikas* to provide treatment. Technical competence proved to be just one consideration; motivating patients and *shebikas* to complete the 12-month course required additional mechanisms. BRAC implemented a contract to explicitly acknowledge that both the patient and the *shebika* had responsibilities. So while the bond ensured patient accountability, the patient was empowered to hold the *shebika* accountable for providing adequate support. The *shebika* was further incentivized by the compensation she received when a patient was cured. BRAC tested this model on the small scale for several years to evaluate whether this model could reliably produce high cure rates and low levels of non-adherence. Then, it expanded the pilot to see if the model could be managed at a larger scale. *Shebikas* needed intensive local support and supervision. As the program grew, central office staff would be unable to provide it themselves and local sources would be increasingly important. In addition, the phase two pilot gave the team time to collect and analyze more data, gaining internal confidence and allowing for broader dissemination. As the global community was slowly regaining its interest in combating TB and gaining appreciation for what would eventually be called directly observed therapy, short-course (DOTS), BRAC's experience demonstrated empirically that these concepts could not only be effectively applied in a low-income country setting, but that they could be conducted at the community level. International support would prove important once BRAC began to think about scaling up nationally and needed to reach out to the public sector.

Chapter 4

Taking the TB Program to Scale in Rural Bangladesh

"Within BRAC, there were never two minds about scaling up TB. There was a demand. We knew that we had to scale up the program. It was deeply ingrained in our thinking that we had to move from a pilot to a larger program to see the effect, believing firmly in 'small is beautiful but taking to scale is essential.' So the program had to move forward."

Sadia Chowdhury, World Bank, formerly BRAC

4.1 Creating a strategy

By 1994, BRAC was eager to expand the TB program. Tuberculosis had become a priority of the global community, and there was significant interest domestically and abroad about programs that could produce high levels of adherence through use of the directly observed therapy, short course (DOTS) strategy (for more information on the DOTS strategy, see Appendix A). BRAC's program had illustrated the power of this approach in rural communities in Bangladesh since 1984. Satisfied with the model and its capacity for managing the program, BRAC now turned its attention to the millions of other rural inhabitants in Bangladesh that lacked access to TB treatment. What strategy would allow BRAC to scale most effectively, quickly, and within its resource constraints?

From its recent experiences with the Oral Therapy Extension Program and scaling up the essential health care program, BRAC had already begun to build a substantial cadre of community health workers on which it could draw. However, financial resources were the first consideration. Most of the TB program's activities could be integrated with other health activities, which made the additional costs fairly minimal. The medications and the laboratory supplies were the largest dedicated expense. In addition, while BRAC had run its own laboratories during the expanded pilot, it had doubts about trying to scale up these activities nationally.

BRAC was aware of the government's plans to scale up facility-based TB services. BRAC believed that it could extend services to the village level while leveraging the government's clinical and laboratory infrastructure. Partnering with the government for large-scale program also seemed important symbolically to avoid duplication and promote program sustainability.

4.2 Public sector activity

Satisfied with the DOTS programs it had implemented in the four sub-districts, the National Tuberculosis and Leprosy Control Program (NTP) decided to scale up nationwide. The World Health Organization (WHO) issued the first international guidelines on DOTS in 1993, and the local team in Bangladesh worked to create guidelines for the national program to endorse. "We visited the fields and worked to get the guidelines together as quickly as we could. There would be a *hartal* [politically supported/enforced strike] going on, and we'd be sitting in a canteen or hotel writing the documents together" Khurshid, WHO, recollects. In late 1993, the government officially adopted DOTS as its national strategy. The World Bank and the government of the Netherlands provided grants for the program to establish DOTS programs in all sub-district facilities over the next four years (Chowdhury and Chowdhury, 1997).

The NTP saw that there were limitations to what the sub-districts' health facilities could provide. Often staff were already overwhelmed with their existing responsibilities. Furthermore, the public health system was largely an impossible option for rural populations who lived far away and could not come for daily treatment. The World Bank had conducted several onsite assessments and recommended that the TB program engage NGOs, such as BRAC, in service delivery.

4.3 Early dialogue

For many years, several NGOs implemented leprosy control services in partnership with the government. Leadership at the NTP believed that a similar model of NGO-government collaboration could be effective for TB control as well. Ahsan Ali, NTP, commented, "BRAC had been informally working at our side for a number of years. In that sense, they were part of the program already, but we wanted to make that official." He met with leadership from BRAC to discuss the potential of a partnership agreement.

Ahsan became an important advocate for BRAC, especially in designing the partnership. Sadia Chowdhury, at BRAC during these discussions, explains, "By having the national program office and its key staff engaged from the get-go [of our TB program], a lot of the people who might have been obstacles to the partnership turned out to be our supporters. We knew then that for a program like this to be scaled up, it would require a very receptive government who agreed that BRAC's involvement would bring value and is enthusiastic about the partnership. They have to believe that your organization's contribution will be an added value to the government's effort and program outcomes." Vikarunnessa Begum, who was at the time with National TB and Leprosy Control Program, shares, "The TB Control Service's resources for scale up were limited, so it thought to engage NGOs, but only those that already had experience in these areas. We had supported the Manikganj pilot and visited it several times. We knew the program well and saw that BRAC had the experience of running a TB program."

BRAC was the first NGO to begin discussions with the government about a partnership for TB control. The issue of the patient bond led to strenuous debate. Ahsan recalls, "Treatment was free, and we did not like the idea of BRAC taking money from the patient. Initially we were quite opposed to it. BRAC explained it to us in another way, emphasizing that they didn't keep the money, that it was more of a contract than a payment. And, that no one would be denied treatment if he couldn't put down a bond." Even representatives from the WHO agreed that, despite the compelling data from the field experiences, the bond created ambiguity in the demarcation between government policy and NGO practice. However, it was one piece of the model on which BRAC refused to compromise, and its leaders backed their decision with their program results: the adherence rate that they were achieving was relatively high, and had only reached that level once the bond was implemented. Eventually the government agreed to allow BRAC to scale up with the bond intact. BRAC agreed to switch from the 12-month regimen that included injections to the new 8-month course recommended in the national guidelines (Figure 4.1).

Sadia says, "It was a very formal process. A memorandum of understanding that was developed and signed between the principles of both parties clearly spelled out exactly what were the roles of the two parties were and what was expected from the government and from BRAC. That document really created a system of accountability for both parties. We had buy-in into this idea of a public-private partnership from the very top of both the Ministry of Health and Family Welfare and BRAC." In April 1994, it was signed by Abed and Ahsan Ali. In addition to the advocacy efforts BRAC and its supporters in the government and WHO conducted, preexisting personal relationships between individuals provided the necessary trust and goodwill to push the agreement through.

4.4 Finalizing the partnership

In internal conversations, BRAC's leaders had roughly estimated that with the government's partnership, they'd be able to expand to 100

Figure 4.1: National treatment guidelines for new sputum smear positive cases in Bangladesh, 1994-2004

Treatment component	Protocol
Regimen for intensive phase (2 months)	Isoniazid, pyrazinamide, ethambutol, and rifampicin daily
Regimen for continuation phase (6 months)	Isoniazid and thiacetazone daily

sub-districts.[1] The national program initially asked BRAC to take 130 sub-districts. BRAC agreed, but soon realized that its current funding levels could not support scale of this magnitude. Fortunately, the national program was also concerned about scaling up so quickly and requested that BRAC scale back its plans. It was decided that BRAC would scale up its program to cover just 60 sub-districts (13 million population).

Subsequently, the national program asked the leprosy coordinating committee, comprised of eight NGOs, to become the leprosy and TB coordinating committee and implement TB control services in 126 sub-districts as well (Bangladesh CCM, 2003, 32). The NGOs managed their

---

[1] Each sub-district has a population of approximately 250,000.

activities through a joint steering committee. The Damien Foundation, a Belgian NGO that began treating leprosy in Bangladesh in 1972, played a lead role in these efforts. Md. Abdul Hamid Salim, who had joined in the early 1990s as a medical officer, had seen firsthand the TB patients that came to the outpatient department in search of treatment. By collecting anecdotal evidence from the staff on people in the community that had died from TB, he was able to persuade the senior leaders to begin to treat TB in 1992. Once the memorandum of understanding was signed, Salim became the convener of all the NGOs that participated in the Leprosy Coordinating Committee. As BRAC had signed a separate memorandum of understanding, it was not technically part of the committee. However, it usually sent staff members to attend the committee meetings as well. Beyond these meetings, BRAC had no interactions with the members of the coordinating committee.

Completion of scale up was scheduled for 1998. By that time, the national program hoped to have established TB programs in all sub-district health facilities. No programming was planned for urban areas, whose health programs fell under the jurisdiction of the city corporations rather than the Ministry of Health and Family Welfare.

4.5 Getting started

Collaboration between partners

In 1995, NATAB wanted to hold a regional conference on the DOTS strategy but lacked funding. BRAC saw this as an opportunity to empower other TB stakeholders and create an opportunity to allow other partners to showcase their achievements. It helped NATAB secure funding from the WHO to organize the conference of the Eastern Region of the International Union against TB and Lung Disease (the Union). Many officials from the government of Bangladesh and foreign dignitaries attended. The strides that Bangladesh had taken in implementing DOTS and moving forward with an ambitious public-private partnership were commended.

BRAC felt that as the lone NGO partner not also involved in leprosy control, it was seen as competition from some of the other partners. It hoped that through its public and behind-the-scenes participation of the conference and other coordinating activities, it could improve its relationship with the other partners. The coordinating meetings between all groups proved an opportunity to share operational lessons from the field. Some of the other NGOs were interested in BRAC's use of less skilled persons trained specifically in microscopy diagnostics, outreach sputum collection centers in remote villages, and the community-based service delivery model, and BRAC provided guidance on how they could replicate these activities in their own programming.

Public sector scale-up

The National TB and Leprosy Control Program faced many challenges in their own scale up efforts. Their first priority was to train health providers on TB. Starting with the Director Generals, they worked down to even the union-level facilities.[2] Under the DOTS strategy, *upazila* (sub-district) health facilities were the primary treatment providers. The program designated a medical officer in each district and sub-district level to be the TB officer, and he would receive some additional training. Before launching the program, a site visit was conducted to evaluate the infrastructure. Many laboratories lacked microscopes and needed renovations. The national program also assessed the sites' capacity to store drugs. These findings were discussed at the central level and arrangements made to address them. Once facilities were deemed functional, the supply chain for medications was established and the program could begin.

An important component of early programming was site visits from the central level. National program staff was constantly traveling, regrouping in Dhaka once every two weeks to discuss their observations on the ground. Visits were an opportunity to give real-time training and identify areas where further support was needed.

4.6 Expanding BRAC's TB program

Assembling the team

Akramul remained the focal person of BRAC's TB program. Taking the program to scale would require not only the top-to-bottom familiarity with the program that he had acquired in his various roles, but operational and managerial competence to ensure quality was not compromised. Sadia's confidence in the plans to scale was in part due to her faith in her program manager. "Akramul shouldered a lot of responsibility for program planning and development. He's not a

---

[2] A union is the smallest administrative unit in Bangladesh, consisting of multiple villages.

physician but he has this ability to understand the technical needs of the program, and what it would take to scale this up. He's not afraid to take risks and try new things and strategies, and once he sees what is doable, he knows exactly who he needs to bring in to make the model work. I'm not exaggerating when I say that had it not been for the program-level partnership between Akramul from BRAC, Dr. Ishikawa from RIT, Japan, and Dr. Ahsan Ali from the National TB Program, we couldn't have gone for the whole program at this point."

Jalaluddin, as head of BRAC's field operations, also provided management for the TB program scale up as one of many programmatic responsibilities. BRAC created the positions of dedicated regional manager to provide direct supervision of implementation. In addition, in each sub-district, it posted a staff person to supervise activities and a medical officer to provide quality control and confirm that cases were appropriately diagnosed and treated.

BRAC was approaching sub-district health facilities to begin discussions on how to work together effectively. In some areas, BRAC encountered resistance despite the official endorsement and scope of work documents from the central level. Though BRAC had commitment to the partnership at the highest level, it also needed to generate buy-in at the lowest level to actually make the program function. Many physician sat the government sub-district health facilities had no contact with the NTP and were skeptical of partnership with an NGO. BRAC team members spent time with the sub-district leadership and staff to discuss the program and value of partnership. BRAC's local staff often invited government staff to visit the program with them and instructed the *shebikas* to refer complicated TB cases to the sub-district health complexes. Over time, the newness of the partnership arrangement wore off and a trust in BRAC's program developed among the public providers. In most sub-districts, open dialog and emphasis on the partnership nature of the program was sufficient to create a window for activity.

During its pilots, BRAC had created its own laboratories for diagnostic microscopy. The memorandum of understanding indicated that microscopy would be performed by the laboratories in the sub-district health facilities. BRAC agreed to provide the staff for these laboratories as necessary. Often several steps were required to have a functioning laboratory. BRAC usually began by approaching the sub-district health facility to learn about their capacity. If they were overwhelmed, they would move to the union-level facilities to see if there was one that had the space for a laboratory. In the cases where no suitable option could be found, BRAC would ask for permission to establish a lab in one of its branch office.

The NTP's central office staff rarely visited BRAC's programs, but asked them to present regularly on their activities. NGOs submitted their performance data to the sub-districts and the data were aggregated before being sent to the central level.

Reaching more communities

BRAC 's essential health care and microfinance programs operated in many of its designated sub-districts but only in localities with potential to become financially self-sufficient. BRAC's mandate from the government was to provide TB treatment throughout the sub-district. In some areas, it would have to implement the TB program without relying on the platform of the village organization. In uncovered villages, local BRAC staff chose *shebikas* from the community themselves. Akramul and his team quickly observed that mobilization and case detection rates were stronger where full *shebika* programs existed, and they compensated as much as possible with intensified support and supervision to the other areas, but it was difficult. In addition, these areas lacked the built-in supervision that the microfinance program provided, so there were often delays in BRAC's learning about challenges in the field or caregiver inactivity.

BRAC had initially planned to scale several programs simultaneously, including microfinance and health. However, it found the microcredit space to be more crowded that it had initially anticipated: in many areas, Grameen Bank and ASA had already set up operations and had created groups among poor women.[3] While BRAC's leadership felt that BRAC could likely complement these activities with the *shebika* program, it decided to shift its scale-up strategy to implement the full range of development activities simultaneously in areas where there were no existing services. When it shared the villages with other development organizations, it was aware that it would need to create demand for its positions in order

---

[3] Grameen Bank and ASA are large microfinance organizations in Bangladesh.

to attract the *shebika*. The financial opportunities provided with the basket of health goods was critical, though the women often possessed an internal motivation to help their community as well. BRAC rarely interacted with these other NGOs at the leadership level. "We didn't want to send the message that we were doing things at an institutional level. Taking a community-by-community approach was more consistent with what we were trying to do." Akramul said.

4.7 Financial challenges

By 1998, scale up in the 60 sub-districts was considered complete. That year, BRAC treated over 6,500 cases and had a cure rate of 89% in its sputum-smear positive cases (n=5,509). By establishing local supervision systems and technical staff, BRAC's central TB team was building the capacity for a decentralized system—one which would enable them to scale the program even further as resources became available.

Nationally, 324 sub-districts (70% of the country) had some level of TB control activity. The government provided services in 214 sub-districts and NGOs were the primary providers in 110 sub-districts (Islam et al., 1999). Cure rates were higher in NGO programs than public sector sub-district health facilities (81% compared to 71%) (Islam et al., 1999). The government estimated an average case detection rate of 25% (Islam et al., 1999).

Throughout this period, it was difficult for public and private programs alike to find donors interested in funding large-scale TB control. The NTP faced significant financial shortages at times, which occasionally resulted in stock outs of medications. BRAC and other partners limited their mobilization efforts when drug supplies were low to avoid enrolling more patients than could be treated.

In 1998, the Bangladeshi government implemented the health and population sector program, which attempted to replace the 126 fragmented and individual projects in a coherent, coordinated effort between the public sector and its development partners, including UN agencies and the World Bank. While overall this restructuring allowed the Ministry of Health and Family Welfare to operate much more efficiently, the World Bank support for the NTP terminated in 1998, decimating the program's resources, and no additional public funds were offered to compensate. Budgetary constraints largely precluded monitoring and supervision. The NTP struggled to maintain the medication supply with smaller grants from donors including the United Kingdom's Department for International Development (DFID), the Canadian International Development Agency (CIDA), and the World Bank.

4.8 BRAC: Internal shifts and scaling up

Towards the end of 1997, Akramul left for Japan to pursue a PhD in public health. He wrote his thesis on the cost-effectiveness of BRAC's community-based TB model in comparison to the sub-district health facility programs supported by the NTP (Islam, 1999). In his absence, Akram Hossain ran the program until he received an opportunity to pursue a master's in public health abroad, at which point Hamidah Hossain assumed the position. Akramul returned in 2000 as BRAC's TB Program Specialist, and Hamidah matriculated in a public health program at Johns Hopkins. With Akramul back at the helm, Abed and two of BRAC's senior advisors, Jon Rohde (formerly UNICEF India) and Richard Cash (Harvard University), decided it was time to implement the program at an even greater scale. BRAC then signed an updated memorandum of understanding increased BRAC's area from 60 to 126 sub-districts (31.5 million population). BRAC requested the opportunity to expand to "low performing sub-districts," ones where large proportions of the population were considered hard-to-reach. As a result, much of its new territory was in the low-lying coastal areas and the Chittagong hill tracts, where the majority of Bangladesh's non-Bengali populations resided. The hill tracts were ethnically diverse, with several distinct languages, and since independence had experienced political oppression and very limited infrastructural development. BRAC was expected to find its own resources for expansion to the 66 new sub-districts.

Generally, BRAC found scale up increasingly easier over time. As the National TB Program expanded its services to all sub-district facilities, training staff and increasing technical capacity, and the newness of the NGO-government partnership wore off, BRAC no longer confronted the same levels of skepticism and wariness from local government officials. In addition, many of the government officials that BRAC had interacted with over the years had been transferred or received promotions from other districts, and greeted BRAC as a familiar partner.

4.9 Emerging needs of a large organization

Structural changes

As described in Chapter 3, BRAC's health program was divided into the health and population division and the rural development program, which managed the essential health care program. Since 1991, TB activities had been included in the health and population division as part of the package of services implemented under the women's health and development program. With the combination of waning funds for TB control and the plans for an extensive scale up, it was integrated with the essential health care program in 1995. Sitting within this structure would allow the TB team to take advantage of rural development program's community presence, supervision systems and existing scale. Though this had always been the long-term plan for successful grant-funded activities, the TB control was more difficult to integrate into the essential health care program than anticipated. The essential health care program's leanness created challenges for maintaining the high levels of support that were required for TB control. Along with some of the other programs expanding at the time, the TB program demonstrated the need for rearrangement and growth in BRAC's organizational structure. Lack of coordinated central supervision decreased accountability in the field—for example, program organizers that supervised *shebikas* did not include any measure of their activity related to TB in their assessment. *Shebikas* often still performed their TB-related responsibilities because they were interested in the remuneration, but their program organizer did not necessarily encourage or know about them, creating the potential for inconsistency and the risk of poor quality services.

In turn, the rural development program's field staff were faced with a new set of responsibilities related to TB control. Program organizers, on top of their existing duties, were expected to nurture new relationships with *upazila* health facilities, establish labs and quality control mechanisms, support supply chain and logistics management, and supervise a revised scope of activities for *shebikas*. These challenges were compounding by the difficulties BRAC found in finding sufficient quantities of good program organizers at the speed that they wanted to scale up. Having adopted the strategy of working primarily through the government laboratories, BRAC also needed to support public sector sub-district health facilities by providing extra staff in overwhelmed laboratories, procuring equipment, and creating functional laboratories. These activities took time, and at times, created delays in BRAC's targets for achieving scale.

The health and population division and essential health care program faced several management and ideological issues in trying to merge TB control activities and other similar initiatives. Historically BRAC had relied on decision-making process of "self-coordination," whereby conversations and negotiations were utilized instead of hierarchy or rule-based systems. The goal was to promote flexibility and adaptation, but to be effective it required time-intensive middle management and a lot of communication (Lovell, 1991, 133). The head of the rural development program at that time was Aminul Alam, a leading member of BRAC's team that had been involved in the pilot at Manikganj. He knew the program firsthand and could appreciate the challenges facing Akramul in straddling fitting the TB program within the essential health care program's architecture. After many conversations, the directors agreed that the need to merge all health programs under one umbrella, separate from the microfinance portfolio, was clear, though it was a change that would need some time to plan and execute. In the meantime, the TB program made some incremental changes to improve the program in the short term. One such action was to create some program organizer positions that were dedicated to tuberculosis programming. Constant dialog between the teams also helped improve relationships and coordination. The TB program found that having its own program organizers was a critical improvement to establishing the program.

In 2003, BRAC moved all health activities into a permanent "BRAC health program" to create greater coordination and efficiency in its growing health portfolio.

Operational adjustments

Human resources

Some modifications had to be made in terms of staffing related to the TB program. At the frontlines, activities were fully integrated into the *shebika*'s package of activities. At the central level, some dedicated staff were needed to ensure overall program quality. In particular, the program increased the number of technical staff at the central and district level to provide guidance, monitoring, and supervision.

In the pilot phases, BRAC had often had one lab technician covering a full one sub-district and practiced quality assurance by conducting occasional peer reviews of a few slides. As scale up led to multiplying demands, peer reviews ceased to be feasible and technicians handled their catchment area independently. Additionally, while NTP guidelines and BRAC's operating procedures instructed programs to use three slides as the basis for their diagnosis, some government facilities lacked the capacity to examine three slides for each patient, so diagnosis were made based on fewer sputum examinations.

> **Selected RED studies conducted during the scale up**
> - A follow up of the community-based TB control program of BRAC
> - The forgotten disease: an evaluation of a community-based control program in rural Bangladesh
> - Relapse of TB in rural areas of Bangladesh
> - Reasons for discontinuation of TB treatment provided by BRAC

In hard-to-reach areas, BRAC found vacancy and absenteeism of laboratory technicians at the government health posts to be a significant challenge. In many cases, BRAC was asked to increase their staff and manage the TB laboratories themselves in addition to their field-level activities.

Expansion efforts were hampered by high levels of turnover among *shebikas*. In 1996, BRAC did an in-depth analysis on *shebika* activity and found a program-wide dropout rate of over 30% over a ten-year period, with some areas experiencing rates as high as 44% in three years (Khan et al., 1998).[4] The reasons varied, but often related to complaints about the work burden, which took them away from their children and household duties, in proportion to the remuneration, which was lower than expected or the effort required (Khan et al., 1998).In areas with local markets, health facilities or private doctors (qualified or not), these issues were magnified. Lack of acceptance in the community and family also factored into their decisions to quit (Khan et al., 1998). High turnover among *shebikas* undermined progress at every level—village organizations and program organizers were forced to take on the activities until another *shebika* was selected and trained, and field staff were distracted from their primary activities. Mobilization efforts were weaker, the

---

[4] The study categorized *shebikas* as "active" and "dropout". The criteria for "active" were participation in two consecutive refreshers, 15 household visits daily, and participation in two health forums per month.

dropout rates among family-planning clients increased, and distribution of health products fell (Khan et al., 1998).

Real-time data analysis

During scale up, the TB program had an increasing number of villages and patients to consider. Field visits by headquarter staff could no longer serve as the primary mode of supervision, as they couldn't visit all sites with the same frequency. Having good program data in hand and staff with analytical abilities to identify areas of concern was crucial to quickly correcting issues of quality that arose. Whereas to date RED had managed almost all of the data management, during this time period, the health program increased its in-house expertise to enable it to maneuver more dynamically. They continued to consult RED for more in-depth questions of evaluation, but recognized that RED's methods of inquiry were better suited for deeper analyses than emergent operational issues requiring immediate attention.

4.10 Looking ahead

In 2001, changes in the national procurement system led to shortages of TB drugs (Bangladesh CCM, 2005, 107). The NTP approached several donors in an attempt to procure the recommended regimen. Again, NGOs were careful to limit their case finding in attempts to avoid enrolling more patients than the program had the current medication supply to treat for the full course.

The partnership had achieved a cure rate of approximately 80% nationally. The program estimated that its detection rate for sputum-smear positive cases was less than 35%, and even less capacity to diagnose other types of TB (Bangladesh CCM, 2003, 9). It had established TB programs in all 460 sub-district health facilities, had 44 chest clinics to handle complex cases, and on average had one diagnostic microscopy facility per sub-district.[5] Most programs had no quality assurance mechanisms and lacked staff with adequate microscopy training(Bangladesh CCM, 2003, 47).

In 2002, CIDA provided technical and financial support to NTP, enabling it to purchase six vehicles to begin supervision efforts. DFID also provided a year's supply of TB medications.

---

[5] The WHO recommends one microscopy center per 100,000 population. Bangladesh's ratio was closer to 1 per 270,000 population.

Internationally, there was increasing interest in strengthening TB control efforts in developing countries. BRAC predicted that the availability of funds would soon increase drastically. In 2002, they approached the government to discuss the remaining uncovered sub-districts. They had recently completed a study that compared the cost effectiveness of its community-based DOTS model with a facility-based program. It showed that though the programs had similar cure rates, per patient

> "Before, we'd never really been under any real pressure to scale. It was more of a 'let's do as much as we think we can' situation. With FIDELIS, there was a lot of flexibility in terms of how we could use the money, but there were specific targets and time parameters. This forced us to work backwards—if we are going to achieve these things within one year, how quickly do we need to make things happen? We saw that we had to get moving. It was really good preparation for the Global Fund."
>
> *Akramul Islam, BRAC*

operational costs in BRAC's program were US $64 compared to US $96 for facility-based programs at the sub-district and district levels (Islam et al., 2002). Upon learning this, the NTP was eager to increase the scale of BRAC's model as a strategy for increasing the overall cost effectiveness of the program.

By 2003, all the sub-districts had an NGO partner supporting public sector TB control activities. BRAC was the largest partner, covering 283 of the total of 460 sub-districts. In this same year, the Global Drug Facility agreed to provide about 50% of TB drugs needed nationally at no-cost through 2005 (Bangladesh CCM, 2003, 34). The increased reliability of the supply chain allowed NGOs to focus their funds on strengthening treatment programming and case detection.

4.11 Experimenting with scale in mind

In the early 2000s, BRAC sought opportunities to scale while maintaining flexibility to answer important operational research questions in the process. In 2003, CIDA provided US $34 million in funding to the International Union against Tuberculosis and Lung Disease (the Union) for the "Funds for Innovative DOTS Expansion through Local Initiatives to Stop TB"(FIDELIS) project. The FIDELIS project was established to provide small operational research grants (US $150,000-250,000) to pilot creative approaches to improving case detection and adherence rates for populations that were often missed by traditional approaches, such as those living in urban slums or remote rural areas. The fund also prioritized supporting local efforts to develop and test solutions. The idea was to enable programs to discover innovative strategies that could then be scaled up and incorporated into practice more broadly (in projects supported by other donors).

BRAC applied for FIDELIS funding in 2003 to test ways to improve its rural TB program. Its proposed strategies included increased engagement of community leaders, religious ones in particular, and using program funds to pay the *shebika* so that the patient received his full bond at the completion of treatment. Similar to the resistance BRAC had encountered with the NTP and WHO, the Union had concerns about how a bond could limit access to care, particularly for the poor. I.D. Rusen, the Union, recalls,

> "We were torn a bit, because we really believe that TB diagnosis and treatment has to be free. There was a concern between having patients put forward a bond, and yet BRAC had demonstrated anecdotally that the patients didn't mind putting the bond forward. And, if a patient didn't have enough, they wouldn't be excluded because BRAC would ask the community to pay. On the flip side, when we reviewed the application, we also had to think about the implications the study would have on the program's sustainability: If BRAC switched to paying the *shasthya shebika*, we had to raise questions about where the funding for the payment would come from when the FIDELIS project ended. At first perhaps the Global Fund dollars would cover it, but what about when that ended. Would the government be able and willing to pay the *shebikas*?"

In 2004, BRAC received FIDELIS funds and expanded to 45 sub-districts, reaching over 15 million more people. Later that year, FIDELIS gave BRAC an additional grant to pilot the *shebika*-based DOTS program in urban and peri-urban areas, which it implemented in a catchment area of about 8 million and demonstrated good results (Bangladesh CCM, 2005, 81). In 2005, FIDELIS extended the grant for rural implementation to enable BRAC to continue its expansion to more sub-districts, and in 2008, extended it again to bring the programming to low-performing areas in the Chittagong hill tracts to cover a population of close to 28 million.

4.12 New dollars for TB: Creation of the Global Fund

In 2002, galvanized by Kofi Annan's call for an international effort to tackle key diseases worldwide, the Global Fund to Fight AIDS, Tuberculosis, and Malaria (Global Fund) was launched. It emphasized country leadership and ownership, calling on countries to create a country coordinating mechanism (CCM), which developed one proposal for the country with its own targets and metrics. The proposal specified the principal recipients, who managed the funds in-country and sub-contracted to all in-country parties. Notably, the Global Fund did not guarantee full funds at the time when a proposal was accepted. Instead, it released funds only when grantees demonstrated achievement of targets and indicators that the countries include in the initial proposal (Elridge and Palmer, 2009). Funds were meant to match the speed of implementation, rather than a fixed calendar. Thus, increases and decreases in disbursements would be made based on past expenditure (Low-Beer et al., 2007).

For those working on what had been an unglamorous disease, the Global Fund signified an influx of resources that had previously been unimaginable. Bangladesh established a CCM in February 2002. It submitted an application in 2002 (Round 2) that did not receive funding. Some attributed this to Bangladesh's relatively limited experience in applying for grants of this type. "We were thinking so narrow," Salim, KNCV TB Foundation, formerly Damien Foundation, remembers, "We framed the question as: if you look at your current programs, what are the gaps? Some programs said that they had none; one NGO said that they needed a single computer. It wasn't until we reframed the question to be, what do you want to be doing? That was when we really started to think big enough to write a strong proposal." There were also some signs made that the Global Fund would be more amenable to a proposal that split the duties of the principal recipient between two institutions to ensure management and absorptive capacities. Marijke Becx, who had worked in Bangladesh for many years, joined the process as an external consultant for the subsequent round. In 2003 (Round 3), Bangladesh applied with two principal recipients. The Ministry of Health and Family Welfare was the first principle recipient and would be responsible for policy creation, guidelines, best practices, and documentation, and BRAC would serve as the second principal recipient, overseeing all service delivery on the part of the NGOs. With technical guidance from the WHO, this arrangement was seen as ideal for several reasons: it would split the management responsibilities, encourage effective division of tasks, and enhance accountability. "While now there are extensive selection criteria for choosing a principal recipient, at that time it was quite simple. BRAC covered more sub-districts than any other NGO, so we chose them as the principal recipient." In the proposal, the CCM wrote that two principal recipients would enable "efficient disbursement, rapid implementation, and greater transparency, for effective utilization of the GFATM fund (Bangladesh CCM, 2003, 122)."

Some of the other NGOs expressed reluctance to become sub-recipients of BRAC, especially as they'd had prior experience coordinating as the Leprosy and TB Coordinating Committee. The creation of the NGO steering committee, which would provide a forum for implementation issues and input into CCM decisions, offered some consolation to the other partners.

In 2004, Bangladesh received an initial grant for US $42.5 million over 5 years (Table 4.1). The agreement was signed in July and US $6.8 million was provided for the first year of programming (NTP, 2005). BRAC handled the sub-contracts to all NGOs. By August, BRAC had disbursed funds for implementation, and in September, implementation using Government of Bangladesh Global Fund funds began.

Table 4.1: Grants received by Bangladesh from the Global Fund for TB control (in US $ millions)

Round	Years of funding	Total funding received	Funding received through NTP as PR	Funding received through BRAC as PR	Number of SRs
Round 3	2004-2009	42.47	15.45	27.02	10
Round 5	2006-2011	49.19	26.45	22.74	29
Round 8	2009-2014	77.08	36.23	40.85	44
Round 10	2011-2016	98.54	51.29	47.25	45
Total funding	2004-2016	267.3	129.42	137.86	

Note: PR=principal recipient. Figures include all money sub-contracted to other partners within Bangladesh.

SR=sub-recipient. Receive funding through a principal recipient. BRAC is both a principal recipient and a sub-recipient.

When the funding disbursements began in 2004, NTP found that it lacked the capacity and experience to manage its funds directly. It asked the WHO to manage its share of Global Fund funds while it improved its internal system. In order to receive Global Fund approval, the WHO had to sign an agreement with the government. This procedure required the participation of several ministries, included the Ministry of Finance and Law, delaying disbursement by over six months.

4.13 From breadth to depth

Prior to receiving the Global Fund's support, Bangladesh claimed to have achieved 100% access to DOTS by its own definition of one facility with TB services per sub-district. However, for most patients, receiving daily treatment from these facilities would be impossible. There were clear areas for expanding quality and access. "In theory, geographical coverage was 100% before Bangladesh received funds from the Global Fund." Salim, KNCV TB Foundation, formerly Damien Foundation, shared. "But we knew that within the geography, much could be done to improve access and strengthen services."

One of the NTP's first priorities was increasing the availability of microscopy centers at the sub-district level and creating a mechanism for external quality assurance. In addition, it strengthened the supply chain and procurement procedures to prevent stock outs at the facility level. With Global Fund dollars, the regimen was upgraded to better match international guidelines.

In order to increase the case detection rate, NGOs needed to strengthen the community component of their programming. Many surveys demonstrated that the social stigma around TB created delays in seeking treatment, particularly in women (Karim et al., 2009). Before receiving support from the Global Fund, communication activities, where they existed, were local and limited. BRAC received support to develop behavioral communication change materials. Soon, they had developed TV and radio spots that were aired on national stations. In addition, they distributed half a million posters and a million stickers with information about symptoms and treatment for TB.

In 2005, with another grant from FIDELIS, BRAC also experimented with many new forms of community mobilization, from popular theatre performances to programs in primary schools. For the first time, BRAC provided orientations for imams (Islamic clerics), Muslim leaders, and cured patients, urging them to act as active case finding agents in their communities. BRAC found that in these areas with the additional mobilization activities, case detection rates increased by 29%, compared to areas without these activities (Rifat et al., 2008).

While some mechanisms had been established centrally to coordinate efforts, at the district and sub-district levels, there were far fewer resources to support collaboration. As a result, capacity and coordination varied widely between partners and within geographies. The National Anti-tuberculosis Association of Bangladesh (NATAB) received funding to revive its district committees and hold regular meetings with civil society. Membership consisted of many traditional stakeholders, including NGO and Ministry of Health and Family Welfare staff, as well as a diverse range of civil society representatives, such as lawyers, teachers, scout leaders, business owners, and leaders of women's groups. These meetings helped create local mobilization and strengthen advocacy for public resources. In addition, as local authorities grew more knowledgeable about TB and understanding of what high quality services entailed, they were better equipped to monitor the programs in their facilities.

Intensifying service delivery

While these efforts could support individuals in seeking treatment, case detection also required measures to make services more accessible. NGO partners experimented with different strategies to improve their rates. For example, BRAC focused on replicating its *shebika* program in more villages within its designated sub-districts.

"Over the years, we had thought of many ways in which the program could be strengthened, but without the resources, they were just ideas. The great thing about the Global Fund was that suddenly there was a mechanism to implement them. So we could move quickly because we knew what we wanted to do," Jalaluddin, BRAC, explains. BRAC's other departments also understood the opportunity that these new resources presented and threw the full weight of the organization behind the scale up effort. Aminul, head of microfinance, offered Akramul hundreds of microfinance program organizers, whose experience enabled them to hit the ground running. These larger institutional resources propelled the scale up significantly.

NGOs took different strategies to improve case detection rates and treatment outcomes. For example, the Damien Foundation sought to leverage the existing informal health system for TB services. It approached village doctors to sensitize them to TB control efforts. While it did not pay them to provide services, it offered a signboard with their name advertising them as a DOT provider, as well as containers, prescription pads and other useful office supplies. Almost 20% of its cases were referred from village doctors (Salim et al, 2006). In addition, the Damien Foundation formalized programs to engage cured patients in case detection. By 2005, it was holding about 700 meetings per year and engaging 21,000 participants. These programs were highlighted by the NTP as a best practice and other NGOs emulated the initiative in their own programming.

From conversations with its field staff, BRAC found that diagnostics were still a significant challenge in many hard-to-reach areas. Individuals with suspected cases of TB found accessing the laboratories challenging. In other places, BRAC used outreach sputum smearing centers to create convenient access points for villagers and decided to expand the strategy. With another grant from FIDELIS, BRAC piloted an incentive system whereby local volunteers received a small honorarium for every outreach sputum center that they held in hard-to-reach areas, particularly in the hill tracts.

Increasing the cure rate for treatment required services that were convenient and supportive. BRAC felt that its *shebika* model and bond system had demonstrated significant value in achieving high levels of adherence. When the FIDELIS-funded study showed that cure rates increased when patients received their entire bond at the completion of treatment, BRAC made this practice standard and paid *shebikas* out of the Global Fund grants.

4.14 Program achievements

National case detection rates and the cure rate increased once Global Fund support began, jumping from 34% and 84% in 2002 to 70% and 92% in 2010, respectively (NTP, 2010; NTP, 2011). Bangladesh adopted a six-month regimen with rifampicin included in the full course (Figure 4.2). In addition, the infrastructure to support the program also increased substantially. By 2004, 85% of rural facilities had external quality assurance programs and eight laboratories dedicated to external quality assurance had been established in Bangladesh (Bangladesh CCM, 2005, 72). Akiko Fujiki and her colleagues from the Research Institute of Tuberculosis of Japan trained all laboratory technicians working in external quality assurance and conducted

Figure 4.2: NTP guidelines for new smear positive patients, 2005-2011

Treatment component	Protocol
Regimen for intensive phase (2 months)	Isoniazid, rifampicin, pyrazinamide, and ethambutol daily
Regimen for continuation phase (4 months)	Isoniazid and rifampicin daily
Sputum testing	Test at month 2, 5 and 6

regular refresher trainings and independent monitoring of their quality. Recording and reporting systems were created in the health facilities. Drug and lab supplies were increased significantly. BRAC established over 400 laboratories, including 23 external quality assurance laboratories for monitoring purposes. Many sites sent their medical officers and program organizers for training. Investments were made in improving decentralized systems as well.

4.15 Persistent challenges

When applying for additional funding from the Global Fund in 2005 (Round 5), Bangladesh added TB control in urban areas to its proposal, noting that these efforts were particularly weak, despite the transmission risks that arose from massive amounts of urban poverty. Constructing effective partnerships and programs in these new areas would continue to challenge the partnerships for the coming years (see Chapter 7 for more discussion on urban programs). For example, case detection in rural areas consistently outpaced case finding in the urban areas. Low demand, in both rural and urban areas, was seen as a barrier to increasing utilization of services.

Bangladesh struggled to build capacity for more complex laboratory activities. Despite the increases in microscopy at the district and sub-district level, the National Reference Laboratory still faced an overwhelming burden of routine microscopy requests. As a result, it was challenged to simultaneously perform the duties typically expected of a reference laboratory, such as drug sensitivity testing. In 2011, NTP opened a second reference laboratory in Chittagong, with support from the Global Fund and the United States Agency for International Development (USAID), to better equip the country with capacity for drug sensitivity testing and diagnosis of multidrug resistant (MDR) TB. NGO partners provided significant support in terms of human resources to operate the facility. Despite these growing capabilities, NTP kept the criteria for MDR testing (failure of category II) stringent, recognizing that the country's ability to treat MDR-TB was developing simultaneously, and overwhelming either system could compromise quality, creating risks of extremely drug resistant (XDR) TB.[6]

Larger political and health system issues had implications for TB programming. For example, the high level of turnover among medical officers in rural areas required the NTP to conduct frequent trainings to ensure that local staff was knowledgeable about the program. Additionally, transfers at the leadership levels were common, and the tenure of the NTP Line Director was often under one year. Many times the Line Directors were transferred from other departments and were unfamiliar with the program. As a result of the Global Fund (GF), TB was relatively well-resourced for Bangladesh, so even those appointees who had previous leadership experience were often unprepared to manage such a large program. These transfers made it difficult to plan and execute a longer-term strategy, and despite issues raised by the Global Fund about this policy, the Ministry of Health and Family Welfare had yet to address the long-term placement of a NTP program manager and line director.

4.16 Accounting for scale

The TB program's ability to achieve scale with these outcomes is in large part due to its integration with BRAC's larger infrastructure. Despite the massive increases on the financial side relative to the TB program, for BRAC's finance office, they were relatively small compared to the overall US $206 million budget that it managed. Akramul and his team could focus on getting the technical aspects of the program in place because that accounting infrastructure was there to support them.

Within a matter of months, TB went from not having its own dedicated budget with BRAC's health program to receiving the FIDELIS funding and becoming a principal recipient of a multimillion dollar grant from the Global Fund (Figure 4.3). Moreover, it was expected to scale up its programs on the ground in parallel. Managing these

---

[6] The Bangladesh National TB Program defines category II as a previously treated smear-positive case, including relapse, treatment after interruption, or treatment failure.

Figure 4.3: BRAC's TB program budget, 2003-2010

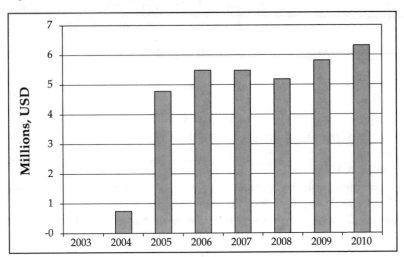

activities required significant organization and strategy at the leadership level to ensure that activities could be carried out by regional and sub-district staff with the appropriate level of independence and standardization. BRAC needed to hire new staff, both technical and financial, for the TB program to manage these increasing responsibilities.

4.17 Trade-offs in scaling up

Akramul was prepared for an intense scale-up phase and communicated to his staff the importance of meeting the targets. He trusted them to determine the most effective strategies for success. One lesson for Mahfuza Rifat, who at the time led trainings for BRAC's TB program, was that it was possible to combine the process of quality improvement and scale up. "In my previous jobs, we'd spent a lot of time making sure the model was right before moving beyond the pilot. Here, I had to start doing trainings almost immediately, so I built a basic curriculum and then worked to improve it over time. In a lot of ways, this embedded the idea of quality being a continuous process, versus just something you think about before scaling up."

The relationships that BRAC had been fostering with public sector staff at the sub-district levels played a critical factor in enabling the pace of scale up that BRAC needed to achieve in order to keep with its targets. In most new sub-districts, BRAC could count on already having worked with a few officials in other places and begin working on implementation almost immediately.

The existing village organizations platform also facilitated rapid scale up. In these areas, BRAC simply needed to work with the village organization to choose a *shebika* and begin the process of training and supervision. In other cases, the *shebika* program already existed but without the TB component. BRAC would work to integrate the additional training and support systems into the health program.

The bigger challenge, however, came from the TB program's mandate to cover an entire sub-district. Since the microfinance program only chose villages with a certain threshold of borrowers, in other villages the program would be implemented without the backbone and supportive mechanisms of the village organization. In these areas, BRAC field staff visited villages and found volunteers themselves, using the existing criteria as a guide.

Though no formal evaluation was ever conducted to see if TB control performance was affected by the presence of a village organization, BRAC's managers observed that without the microfinance platform, the program required much more program support. Anecdotally, *shebikas* without the village organizations were much more likely to drop out, and it took BRAC more time to become aware of their inactivity, as they lacked strong relationship with these communities that existed in places with village organizations. The ordering of the activities mattered as well; the TB program should be built on the village organization, not vice versa. An unanticipated issue arose when the microfinance arrived: the dynamic differed from areas where the *shebika* emerged from the village organizations. In many cases, existing *shebikas* did not want to join the village .organizations. BRAC opted to stick with its criterion of village organization membership as part of the selection process, and in these cases, would choose a new *shebika* to serve the community.

Inspiring the team

As the TB program grew, Akramul knew that he would need a strong set of managers across the program to maintain its quality. He implemented several strategies to build these capacities in his team, both at the central level and in the field. Many had strong technical backgrounds already, but they were encouraged to take advantage of available training opportunities. High-performing field staff were often invited to trainings offered by BRAC or the NTP as recognition of their accomplishments. BRAC tried to bring in international experts to train staff and invited visitors to see these programs firsthand, guided by local program organizers and junior head office staff. These opportunities cultivated a sense of pride and ownership in local staff that inspired commitment to the program. Media advocacy activities often had a similar effect, as they gave field staff a chance to share the program with local elites, creating opportunities for recognition of their activities.

"When you give people something to read, they never find the time. But if you ask them to write something or to present on something, then they have to read in order to get the information," said Akramul. All members of the headquarters staff were given opportunities to develop grant proposals, presentations for meetings and workshops, and submit abstracts or papers to conferences. When local events were held, junior staff were often asked to moderate or record the session. Over time, staff grew comfortable representing BRAC and had more confidence in their interactions with external audiences. Internal dialog was also encouraged; when making program decisions, all staff had an opportunity to share their opinions and participate in the process.

Exposure to other program and international colleagues brought new ideas and energy to the team. BRAC staff participated in regional trainings conducted by the International Union against TB and Lung Disease (the Union), and occasionally staff were able to arrange visits to programs in nearby countries, such as India or Afghanistan. These opportunities were framed as learning experiences that were rewards for a strong work ethic and performance, to create a sense of motivation in the team.

In the past two years, BRAC has begun to bring all sub-district managers to Dhaka annually for modular courses developed by the WHO on TB. Managers at all levels are expected to complete two weeks of managerial training at BRAC's training center, as well as coursework on monitoring and evaluation and TB. While the focus of the courses was on the content, BRAC tried to structure these learning opportunities to enable dialog between staff, creating a sense of professional solidarity.

This combination of formal and informal training, continuous dialog, and cultivation of ownership and pride enable the TB program to effectively operate in a decentralized manner with strong management across the board. Partnership with practitioners at the local facilities and chest clinics and hospitals has created local nodes of technical expertise, reducing reliance of central level support for medical issues. National guidelines provide significant programmatic direction as well. The result is an ability to rapidly respond to local challenges and situations.

4.18 Mobilizing resources

In 2010, the Country Coordinating Mechanism (CCM) began to prepare to submit another proposal to the Global Fund (Round 10). Now that the basic services had been established and intensified nationally, and the urban programming was underway, the country could begin to focus on the new generation of urgent issues in TB control, such as achieving universal coverage for TB care. The proposal included plans to scale up diagnosis and treatment services for multidrug resistant TB, sputum smear negative and extra-pulmonary TB, childhood TB, and lung health.

In this proposal, the CCM also included findings from recent research studies and incorporated them into recommendations for practice nationwide. For example, with FIDELIS funding, BRAC had tested strategies to increase case detection in sub-districts with low case detection rates, such as increased community-based orientations and incentives to volunteers for holding outreach sputum smearing centers in hard-to-reach areas.

4.19 Conclusions

"Scaling an idea requires every bit as much entrepreneurship as piloting one."

David Bornstein and Susan Davis (Bornstein and Davis, 2010)

BRAC's program grew from covering a population of less than two million to over 91 million in the course of sixteen years (Table 4.1). While scale up at times occurred at a heated pace, many of the investments that BRAC made took time to demonstrate their true value. Investing in staff development and relationships across the public health system have some immediate impact, but also a longer-term return on investment in enabling BRAC to react quickly as new opportunities arise. Decentralization requires continuous investment in management systems, but enables a large-scale program with the ability and confidence to act locally as needed. While encouraging a team approach, BRAC was also conscientious about specifying a scope of activities for every team member and providing individual feedback. It found that that the existence of strong role clarity enabled teams to function the most productively.

As the TB program scaled, BRAC grew increasingly conscious of its role in complementing and strengthening the National TB Program. It filled holes in the system when necessary, but avoided building parallel structures or duplicating activities where possible. At times, it was forced to choose between speed of scale up or investment in systems. As is discussed in more depth in the following chapter, the complexity of TB control requires a spectrum of skills that, in a context like Bangladesh, can best be achieved through collaboration between multiple actors. BRAC's greatest strength lay in bringing the basic package to people's doorsteps, and it understood that it could maximize its value by extending and creating bridges to the existing provision of complex clinical services. Engaging local providers and utilizing their expertise also created institutional relationships and decreased reliance on BRAC's central staff. As the public sector's capacity has increased in recent years, for example in strengthening its laboratory system, some of BRAC's earlier activities have subsided. This allows it to focus on new challenges, such as populations that are difficult to reach, or how to engage the immense private sector in the DOTS strategy (see Chapter 7 for more discussion on these activities). Engaging with and learning from other NGOs has proven to be an increasingly important component to effective TB control.

BRAC's evolution at an organizational level also reflects the changes that maturity and scale require. Informal systems and processes allow for rapid prototyping at the pilot phases, but offer minimal enforcement of quality and standardization once a program grows. Information systems, explicit protocols, and intensive supervision systems enable program leaders like Akramul to maintain a comprehensive view of operations from the executive level, and provide the responsiveness infrastructure for program refinements or growth. Despite the increasing bureaucracy and organizational infrastructure, nothing replaces the need for clear communication between the field staff and the central office. Field visits, which help central managers and technical staff appreciate the realities of the field and small-scale innovations, must be maintained, particularly when trying to control a condition like TB that evolves in the rapidly changing context of modern-day Bangladesh. Systems enable individuals to perform efficiently, but they rely on motivated and skilled staff to truly produce stellar results. Creating a culture that instills high levels of productivity, creativity, and commitment requires investment and foresight on the part of leaders and managers.

From scaling up to "at scale"

The term "at scale" has been applied generously and with little precision. While BRAC's strategy is often boiled down to "small is beautiful, but large is necessary," in practice BRAC takes a multifaceted approach to scale. Many experts on scale-up have noted that quantitative scale alone may fail to be sustained without additional mechanisms to support and strengthen these activities. Uvin and Miller have described four types of scale that NGOs can attempt (Uvin and Miller, 1996). While they do not place any judgment on the order that NGOs pursue these different dimensions, in order to maintain value at scale, it may be important for an NGO to have achieved most or all of these. BRAC has incorporated these various domains into its strategy and operations and demonstrates how these can continue to evolve over time.

BRAC started with **functional** scale. It had a small portfolio of development programs, beginning with a strong focus on income generation and microfinance that expanded in scope as it became clear that the drivers of poverty were much more systemic. Often new initiatives were instigated by the communities themselves.

In its Oral Therapy Extension Program, BRAC began to really prioritize **quantitative** scale, expanding the program into areas that did not have the existing platform of economic activities. Based on success in this experiment, BRAC began to expand its health and economic programming more broadly.

When deciding to scale up its TB program, BRAC realized that it lacked the capacity to manage the health system components that would be required to effectively support the front-line community treatment. In a move to create **political** scale, it approached the government to develop a partnership,

(contd.)

(contd.)

therefore promoting government partnership with NGOs and adoption of the DOT strategy in its National Tuberculosis Program. Initially continuing its quantitative scale up to 60 sub-districts in Bangladesh, by 2011 BRAC covered 297 sub-districts.

As the Global Fund was launched, BRAC became one of the principal recipients of funding for TB activities in Bangladesh. It began to provide training and technical support to other NGOs to expand and improve the availability and quality of TB services beyond its own direct catchment areas, all examples of **organizational** scale. Through working meetings and other types of collaborative engagements, it aims to strengthen partnerships across NGOs and with the public sector.

In recent years, BRAC has shifted the focus of its TB programs from expansion to refinement. Realizing that TB was diagnosed much more often in men than women, it undertook operational research to learn whether this trend was indicative of epidemiological patterns or uneven case finding. Front-line staff members were supported in strengthening efforts to access women and the gender disparity has almost disappeared. In the urban areas in particular, BRAC has been active in determining ways to increase its case finding rate and improve treatment adherence among patients.

BRAC has additionally begun to increase its TB programming in the urban areas, creating new models with private partners. Pressure from communities to launch programs targeting malaria and maternal and child health have led to new lines of services.

Types of scale are interconnected, and large organizations must consider these dynamics in their planning. During its early years, BRAC lacked field knowledge to expand horizontally; concentrating its efforts locally allowed it to steep its staff in the programming and gain a deep knowledge of village dynamics, local needs and priorities, and hidden innovations. As this knowledge bank grew, quantitative expansion grew more feasible and with increasing speed. BRAC has been quite deliberate about its interactions with Bangladesh's government, remaining as neutral as possible to the inter-party competition. However, to function in such a wide geography, BRAC needs the legitimacy of the public sector to operate effectively. Partnership with the government offers technical benefits, but also is central to BRAC's philosophy of building a better Bangladesh.

Table 4.2: Timeline on BRAC's activities in TB

Year	BRAC in Bangladesh	BRAC International
1972	BRAC founded	
1977	*Shasthya shebika* and *shebok* pilot initiated in Manikganj	
1980	The oral therapy education program launched	
1984	TB program piloted in Manikganj	
1990	First TB pilot concluded	
1991	Women's health and development program begun; includes second TB pilot expanded to 10 sub-district	
	BRAC TB publishes first article on Manikganj experience	
1994	Bangladesh adopts DOTS as national strategy	
	Conclusion of second TB pilot	
	Memorandum of understanding signed with NTP to implement services in 60 sub-districts	
	BRAC adopts 8-month regimen in line with NTP guidelines	
2001	BRAC signs new memorandum of understanding with the NTP to increase its coverage to 106 sub-districts	
2002	BRAC increases its coverage to 126 sub-districts	BRAC establishes presence in Afghanistan
2003	Cadre of *shasthya kormi* introduced BRAC receives first grant from FIDELIS	BRAC begins to implement the basic health package in Afghanistan
	BRAC increases its coverage to 283 sub-districts	*Shasthya kormi* role conceived and implemented˙
2004	Bangladesh receives first grant from the Global Fund for TB control; BRAC serves as principal recipient for the 10 NGO partners	
	BRAC increases its coverage to 283 sub-districts	
2005	National TB Program adopts 6-month treatment regimen for new smear-positive cases	Afghanistan incorporates facility-based DOTS in the basic health package of services

(contd.)

(Table 4.2 contd.)

Year	BRAC in Bangladesh	BRAC International
2006	Bangladesh receives another grant from the Global Fund for TB control; BRAC now manages 27 partners	BRAC establishes programs in Uganda and Tanzania BRAC Afghanistan received funding from FIDELIS for community-based TB services
2007	BRAC wins Kochon prize for TB program	BRAC establishes program in Southern Sudan
		Afghanistan adds community-based DOTS to national TB guidelines
2008		BRAC establishes programs in Sierra Leone and Liberia
2009	Bangladesh wins another round of funding from the Global Fund for TB control; BRAC is the principal recipient for 41 NGO partners	BRAC Afghanistan becomes sole principal recipient of Global Fund resources for TB control
2010		BRAC Haiti established
		BRAC Uganda pilots TB program
2011	BRAC's coverage increases to 297 sub-districts	
	44 NGO partners involved in TB control	

Chapter 5

Joining Forces: A Public-Private Partnership for TB Control

"If you want to go fast, go alone. If you want to go far, go with others."

African proverb

In many of its health projects, BRAC had informally partnered with the government to achieve better results. As early as the 1970s, BRAC's paramedics had mobilized communities and supported them in accessing government services and assisted in vaccination campaigns. For TB, beginning in 1994, BRAC and the National Tuberculosis Program (NTP) formalized their relationship to enable coordination on a large scale. By this point, the government was quite familiar with BRAC and there was significant trust in their commitment to furthering the public sector's objectives. However, few donors had great interest in a program dedicated to TB in the 1990s, so BRAC's scale up was relatively slow. Launched in 2002, the Global Fund to Fight AIDS, TB, and Malaria (Global Fund) represents a surge in dedicated resources for TB. But accessing those resources would require the NTP and the various NGOs working in TB control to develop an active partnership, as the Global Fund would only accept one proposal from the country. New resources meant new opportunities to strengthen programs and systems in ways previously unimaginable, but demanded a new mode of collaborative operation. In 2004, the national partnership for TB control included 10 NGOs, including BRAC, implementing TB control services. In 2011, there are 44 institutions working on TB control, including several non-implementing partners that provide technical support and operational research (Bangladesh CCM, 2009, 41). Management and alignment of partner activities requires leadership, active support and relationship maintenance. In addition, the partnership has to consider how their activities can strengthen the health system on a broader level.

Partnerships have been widely recommended as a strategy for health delivery in developing countries. One of the major motivations is to improve access to health services for underserved populations in the context of constrained resources, potentially while contributing to longer-term efforts to augment capacity for sustainable health service delivery. In addition, the benefits from effective partnerships can include increased attention to health issues on the national agenda and strengthening national health policy processes and content. Partnerships can mobilize additional funding, stimulate research and development, and increase stakeholders' ability to inform international norms and standards (Table 5.1) (Buse and Hamer, 2007). Administratively, partnerships can result in greater absorptive capacity. But partnerships do not inherently provide good results. These areas of potential value creation all

Table 5.1: Application of contribution areas framework to TB control in Bangladesh

Areas of contributions by global health partnerships	Example from TB control in Bangladesh
Getting specific health issues onto national and international agendas	Public sector and civil society jointly developing plans for national TB control
Mobilizing additional funds for issues	Four successful proposals to the Global Fund
Improving access to cost-effective healthcare interventions among populations with limited ability to pay	Case detection rate increased drastically; treatment available at no cost nationally
Augmenting health service delivery capacity	Sub-district health facilities provide DOTS; NGOs implementating per national guidelines
Strengthening national health policy processes and content	Increased coordination and planning between stakeholders in TB and related provides (e.g. HIV)
Establishing national norms and standards	External quality assurance for all laboratories; central supply chain for medications
Stimulation research and development	Prevalence survey and impact studies conducted; drug sensitivity surveillance underway

Source: Buse and Hamer, 2007.

assume the nontrivial task of creation and maintenance of a functional and effective partnership.

Bangladesh's partnership for TB control has made great strides in tackling TB nationally. Its experience and model are illustrative of the investments required and challenges that the approach can present. It is still in the midst of developing additional capacity to control TB and demonstrates the magnitude of the challenges that a developing country with limited functional health system infrastructure faces in tackling a disease. Also, even in the presence of political will and eager NGO partners, some activities take time. We explore these issues here, presenting our current struggles and insights to aid other countries that are similarly engaged with these decisions.

5.1 Roles and responsibilities

As mentioned in the previous chapter, the Global Fund greatly transformed the landscape for development and funding for health. It requires countries to create a body called the Country Coordinating Mechanism (CCM) that represents not just the public sector, but implementing NGOs and other stakeholders in civil society. It inspires a stronger sense of equality between partners—not only does it give them an opportunity to be at the table and participate in decision making. Its accountability measures require that funds get spent (or returned to the Global Fund), and not only spent, but spent as outlined in the proposal. Resources could not be channeled to other health programs or expensive "health systems" purchases. NGOs are still expected to support the public sector strategy and priorities, but all entities now have far higher levels of accountability to each other. Certainly this structure has limitations, but for TB control in Bangladesh, the Global Fund model of aid motivated the many stakeholders that had been working on TB largely in isolation to begin to plan and work together more closely.

All partnerships require an institution that provides strong leadership and a common vision between stakeholders. The NTP is best positioned to lead, but has lacked the consistency of a strong, dedicated director that is crucial for nurturing the partnership. No coordinating body or NGO can fully compensate for the absence of this strong leader from the public sector, with the dedication and equally important length of tenure to truly manage the partnership's

Figure 5.1: Map of Bangladesh by NGO implementing partner, 2010

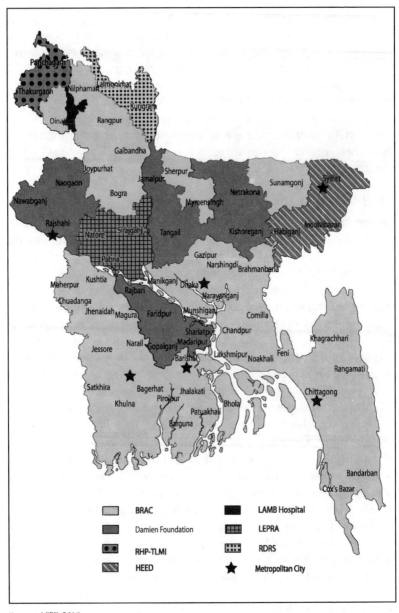

evolution over time. That said, they can create mechanisms to promote collaboration, consistency, and joint action where appropriate.

Members

The National Tuberculosis Program leads the partnership and directs the activities of all other partners. NGOs provide significant support in service delivery and in mobilizing communities to utilize public services. BRAC, as the Principal Recipient, has assumed a contractual relationship with the other NGOs and is mandated to provide supervision and support.

After BRAC, the Damien Foundation is the next largest implementing partner. Together, they account for 80% of national coverage by population (Figure 5.1).The International Center for Diarrheal Disease Research, Bangladesh participates as a research partner.

Coordinating bodies

The Bangladesh Country Coordinating Mechanism (CCM) was established in February 2002. The chairperson and vice chairperson roles are filled by the Honorable Minister and the Secretary of the Ministry of Health and Family Welfare, respectively. The CCM's role is to identify the priority areas from the national disease control strategic frameworks for HIV, TB, and malaria. It dictates the partnership's areas of focus, procedural aspects, and oversees implementation. It must approve the principal recipients. It submits proposals to the Global Fund on behalf of Bangladesh. Its members include the government, NGOs, academic institutions, and civil society groups.

The interventions proposed in the strategic plan for TB control (2011-2015) are:

- Pursue quality DOTS expansion and enhancement
- Establish interventions to address HIV-associated TB and drug-resistant TB
- Contribute to health systems strengthening
- Forge partnerships to ensure equitable access to an essential standard of care for all TB patients
- Engage people with TB and affected communities
- Promote operational research

Source: WHO, 2010, 5.

In addition to the CCM, another entity was established to focus on NGO implementation and facilitate collaboration, called the NGO steering committee. Some of the other NGOs also saw this mechanism as a way of maintaining some additional accountability for BRAC in its dual role of implementer and principal recipient. In addition to the NGOs, the WHO and NTP participate to stay informed on the issues and provide expert input. The steering committee's schedule is not fixed, and the frequency of meetings varies.

Public sector organization for TB control

The NTP sits within the Mycobacterial Disease Control Directorate, whose Director also serves as the Line Director for the TB & Leprosy Program. The Program Manager oversees the NTP operations, with the assistance of three deputy program managers and five medical officers. Historically there have also been high levels of turnover among medical officers, who oversee coordination, procurement, logistics, training, administration and finance.

Implementation and supervision of TB activities is integrated into general health services at the district and sub-district levels. Each of Bangladesh's 64 districts has a civil surgeon, who oversees all Ministry of Health and Family Welfare activities, including TB. Approximately two thirds of districts have a dedicated TB Program Officer or a TB Medical Officer; filling these positions nationally is a persistent challenge (WHO, 2010, 46). The civil surgeon has ultimate authority over TB programming at the district level, and the program officer provides direct support and coordinates meetings.

Within the 483 upazilas (sub-districts), the local Health and Family Planning Officer's responsibilities encompass supervision of the NTP programming. One medical officer focuses on disease control, including TB, and the TB and Leprosy Control Assistant supports him or her in running the sub-district's program. At the union and village level, the Ministry of Health and Family Welfare aimed to provide one domiciliary worker (health assistants, assistant health inspectors, and health inspectors) per five to six thousand population (DGHS, 2010).

5.2 Supervision of partner activities

Strong mechanisms for supervision are critical for effective service delivery, particularly in a large partnership where NGOs are delivering services on behalf of the public sector. Supervision creates accountability for quality standards, allows for rapid identification of gaps in knowledge or resources, and emphasizes public sector ownership of the programs. Ultimately, the NGO partners are responsible to the NTP, and its obligations consequently include supervision. Forms of supervision vary and best results are seen when a combination of activities are implemented. Critical components include onsite supervision, reporting, and review meetings. The NTP has included all of these activities in its plan, with both local and national-level responsibilities.

However, operationalizing robust supervision in the context of a decentralized and integrated service delivery system is challenging. Creating the infrastructure for effective supervision takes time, and often investments at this level only begin after the basic service delivery infrastructure has been erected.

Onsite supervision

The NTP must ensure that NGO partners provide services that are aligned with national guidelines and meet its quality standards. Onsite visits are one of the best strategies for quickly assessing a program's operations. The primary supervisory responsibility falls on sub-district staff. Their proximity allows most frequent communication and convenience of visiting. However, competing responsibilities (including the many not related to TB) often result in postponement of supervisory visits. In 2010, occasional surprise visits made by the sub-district-officer or district medical officer were the major form of local supervision.

NTP staff also try to visit programs at least once a quarter, though other administrative duties can interfere with this schedule. The NTP has developed a supervisory checklist that it uses to organize the activities it conducts on its visits. These include inspecting the laboratory, quality of the slides, completeness and accuracy of the registry, and interviewing patients, when present.

BRAC has additional supervisory responsibilities to the NGOs to which it sub-contracts. It tries to visit all partners on a quarterly basis with a supervisory checklist based on its responsibilities from the Global Fund. In addition reviewing records, clinical, laboratory, and inventory practices, it also reviews financial activity to ensure consistency with performance data. BRAC holds a quarterly meeting with each partner to discuss activity from the prior three months. If any financial irregularities are found, BRAC sends the partner a note and expects an explanation within 30 days. Often the irregularity can be explained by a data error and is easily resolved. If not, BRAC will call a meeting with the partner and if necessary, suspend payments until issues are resolved or the partnership is terminated. BRAC has a zero tolerance policy for corruption and has a separate monitoring department to oversee internal and partner activities on this level (this is discussed in more depth in Chapter 9). Joint supervisory visits ensure clarity of roles, consistency of messages by supervisors, and complete communication of expectations and priorities between all partners. NTP and BRAC have agreed to coordinate on supervisory activities to the extent possible. The current challenge is to create the supervisory capacity at the district and sub-district level. There are some areas where only BRAC is providing supervisory visits on a regular basis (WHO, 2010, 18).

The need for increased supervision is acknowledged internally and in external assessments, such as the 2010 Joint Monitoring Review conducted by the World Health Organization. One finding of the review was that patients often receive weekly drug supplies for self-administration, despite stated the guidelines of directly observed therapy. Supervision itself takes time to institutionalize and implement: local staff must be empowered and required by their superiors (within the NTP and more broadly) to conduct regular supervisory activities. Without adequate training and resources, this is quite challenging. As the NTP and the broader health system continue to increase its staff and infrastructure, BRAC provides some of the basic supervisory roles as required by the Global Fund.

Reporting

Reports are provided on a quarterly basis to the NTP providing information on partner activities in four major categories: case finding, outcomes, sputum conversion, and laboratory findings. These enable the NTP to gauge the performance of partners, identifying low-performing areas that require additional support, and plan for procurement. Joint submission of reports also creates a shared sense of achievements between the public and NGO providers. Sub-district health facility staff coordinate with NGOs to compile a detailed report of all activities. In addition, they collaborate with the staff in the civil surgeon office to consolidate the sub-district reports into aggregated district forms, which are all submitted to the NTP.BRAC also receives a copy of the sub-district reports to enable it to perform its own supervisory activities.

Upazila health complexes maintain paper-based records and submit hard copies to the NTP. At the central level, data is manually entered into the electronic database. Significant time and human resources are therefore required at each level to compile the data and ability to analyze and utilize the data real-time is limited. For example, the NTP currently lacks the capacity to provide feedback on data quality or use the data for corrective measures (WHO, 2010, 19). Plans are underway to move to an electronic system at the sub-district level. In some areas, hardware is now available and staff are trained in doing so. The NTP sees this transition as a critical step in enabling a more responsive and data-driven system, but also wants to move slowly to ensure that the implementation process occurs smoothly, data quality is maintained, and disruptions are avoided as much as possible.

Review meetings

Review meetings provide another mechanism to promote accountability and joint problem solving. They are also an important planning forum to mitigate future risks—for example, reviewing how inventory of laboratory supplies and medication compare to utilization and enrollment rates can ensure that supplies are maintained at appropriate levels. The NTP recommends that the sub-district staff meet with the NGO staff quarterly, and in addition, coordinate a district-level quarterly meeting, where the Civil Surgeon, district program officer, sub-district staff, representatives from the NTP, and NGO representatives review activities and recent reports. These meetings enable the public sector officials to gain a deeper understanding of the NGO's operations and provide support where necessary, if there are ongoing technical challenges.

Currently, meetings at the national level with representatives from the NTP, NGO partners, and WHO occur primarily at the proposal planning stage. Plans exist to instate quarterly meetings to expand coordination, regular planning, and monitoring, as these have not happened regularly in recent years (WHO, 2010, 19). Leaders observe that an active champion of coordination is necessary to catalyze these meetings. Often, the WHO plays this role, as it is well poised to support the NTP in bringing all partners together around these issues.

5.3 Relationships and collaboration

Systems for coordination and collaboration are critical for any partnership. However, in programs for controlling a condition like TB, which must be dynamic and responsive to challenges as they arise, there is no substitute for regular communication. Relationships between institutions and individuals facilitate these conversations and are helpful in finding solutions quickly. One challenge faced by the partnership is balancing the needs for central-level control and local responsiveness. In general, the health system is controlled by national level policy and decision-making. In this context, encouraging local staff to work with NGOs to problem solve locally can be difficult, but waiting for formal endorsement at the central level creates delays. As capacity is built at the lower levels, the NTP continues to evaluate the best strategy for balancing these issues and existing public sector procedures.

In addition, intensity of partnership varies by NGO and sub-district. The Damien Foundation has established centers within the sub-district health facilities, an activity that perhaps does not enable the most rapid initiation of intense service delivery, but one that creates a platform for long term relationship building. BRAC prioritized activities at the community level and built a temporary parallel infrastructure to enable more diagnostics in the short term than the public sector facilities could handle. In recent years, it has focused more on relationships at the local levels and begun to close many of its own laboratories, instead working with the sub-district facilities. However, public sector ownership can take time to cultivate, particularly if local managers see the project as belonging to someone else. In areas where BRAC staff have been particularly proactive, sub-district staff are occasionally reluctant to add the TB activities to their activities. One long-time senior level person in the TB partnership reflected, "BRAC's team was really dedicated and committed to success [of implementation]. There was a marked difference in their commitment from the government staff at that time. As BRAC's program grew, government staff would look on and say, 'BRAC's got it under control. What more do we need to do?'"

BRAC now must be deliberate and proactive in transferring and promoting and strengthening ownership among district and subdistrict staff.

Division of responsibilities

In both the Global Fund contract and individual memorandums of understanding with NGO partners, the NTP articulates the responsibilities for each entity (Table 5.2). For the national program to effectively control TB, both sides must fulfill their obligations. Creating clear expectations allows for accountability on both sides. It also allows partners to focus on their specific tasks, instead of worrying about the whole system. "It's a lot easier for BRAC's district and *upazila* managers to focus on supervising the *shebikas* when they know that they don't have to worry about where the drugs are coming from or monitoring the quality of the lab. Having partners who look after these key pieces of the system enable them to concentrate on doing their job well," says Akramul, BRAC.

While in extreme circumstances these roles may vary, for the most part they are representative of activities nationwide. In areas where the NTP faces particularly severe human resource shortages, NGO partners may increase their responsibilities to compensate.

Table 5.2: Division of responsibilities

Area	Government	NGOs
Health system strengthening and capacity building	National guidelines, technical training, overall coordination	Local training, strengthening of services, performance, civil society involvement
Diagnosis and treatment	Equipment and supplies	Diagnosis, treatment and follow up
Drug supply External quality assurance	Procurement and distribution Training and provision of space	Transportation and distribution Establishment and management external quality assurance laboratories
Monitoring and supervision	Overall monitoring and supervision	Local monitoring and supervision, repoting, annual data validation, audit

Procurement and logistics

Providing medications for the TB program is a core responsibility of the NTP. With over 158,000 patients in 2010, it is critical for procurement to take place in a centralized and efficient manner (NTP, 2011). Importation of medications and laboratory supplies is subject to many customs and administrative procedures; NGOs lack the leverage that the NTP has to ensure that these processes do not threaten the national drug supply. However, even when the public sector assumes this role, it must be vigilant about potential causes of delays and shortages.

The NTP uses program reports to estimate the country's national need to place local and international orders. About 95% of all anti-TB drugs were purchased through the Global Drug Facility, the Stop TB partnership's mechanism that provides access to high quality medications at competitive prices. Until 2008, WHO handled the quantification, procurement, and distribution of non-medicine items while the NTP made efforts to build their internal capacities in these areas. In addition, capacity to store the drugs required acquisition of additional space. In 2009, the NTP acquired an additional storage space and currently employs six full-time staff to maintain inventory of first-line medications and laboratory supplies at the central level (WHO, 2010, 20-21). Second-line drugs are kept separately, at the National Institute of Diseases of the Chest and Hospital. As required by the WHO and Global Fund, these medications are all procured via the Global Drug Facility.

Given the importance of avoiding interruptions in patient treatment regimens, TB medication supply chains must account for all possible areas of delay. For example, delays in funding can lead to inability to get drugs cleared by customs. Vulnerabilities of this type demonstrate the importance of political commitment to TB; secured funds or access to emergency reserves in the case of lacking external dollars is crucial for timely procurement. In addition, additional measures to monitor stock at the central level can also minimize the risk of these issues arising. These can also help the NTP anticipate requests from partners and enable them to replenish their supply quickly, avoiding the need to delay initiation of treatment of new patients. The NTP currently does not have robust measures in place, but hopes to address these issues in coming years.

As the NTP focuses on scaling up its ability to manage a comprehensive supply chain with the appropriate safeguards, NGOs provide support for simple logistics. NGOs like BRAC with significant infrastructure in many hard-to-reach areas can efficiently assist the NTP in moving the supplies and medications in the short-term.

Service delivery

Bangladesh has 64 districts, which further divide into 483 *upazilas* (sub-districts).The public sector and one partner NGO provide services in each sub-district. Each sub-district has a population of approximately 250,000, and one sub-district health center that typically has 30-50 beds is the main public sector provider of DOTS treatment. In addition, there are 9,722 community health clinics providing basic outpatient services.[1] Two thirds of districts additionally has a chest clinic that has the capability of delivering more complex care, such as diagnosis of extra pulmonary TB. While some NGOs provide clinical services, they all coordinate referrals with public facilities to ensure maximum utilization of existing resources.

NGOs agree to provide certain types of services, and the NTP largely considers partner results rather than requiring a specific implementation model. One area where the NTP feels that NGOs have a strong comparative advantage is around community mobilization. The value that a partner like BRAC provides is increased linking of patients with government services, and the extension of government services to communities in a way that the public sector currently lacks the capacity to directly do. In addition to the specifications laid out in the memorandums of understanding and the national guidelines, the NTP discusses the value of creating more stringent guidelines. For example, they currently do not have a definition for "coverage" for NGOs at the sub-district level. In a model like BRAC's, where community mobilization is a key component of the value proposition, the NTP may want to ensure that BRAC maintains an active *shebika* in every village. However, expanding their guidelines will increase the supervision that they are

---

[1] The government plans to establish a total of 18,000 community clinics; one per 6,000 population (DGHS, 2010).

required to provide, so it must move gradually as its own capacity increases.

Engaging village doctors in TB control

The Damien Foundation has 6,100 fixed DOTS centers in its catchment area. One of its strategies to create community demand for TB screening includes cured patient clubs, where staff motivate former patients to mobilize their communities. In addition, the Damien Foundation has had great success in engaging village and medical doctors in voluntarily providing referrals to suspected cases for diagnosis at their facilities. Success is in large part due to substantial efforts to engage village doctors in orientations. In 2010 alone, over 7,000 village doctors participated in trainings.

Sources of referrals, (%)

Year	Cured patients	Govt. health staff	Village doctors	Other
2010	19	35	12	34

Village doctors are important providers of DOTS in their communities. Once a case is diagnosed, a patient can opt to receive treatment under the support of their local village doctor. Currently, over 60% of Damien Foundation patients are supervised by village doctors.

Research

In 2007, two research committees for TB were established, one to focus on technical issues, and the other focused on implementing and monitoring. Several implementing NGOs participate in research activities as well, including BRAC and the Damien Foundation. Cumulatively, the Global Fund has committed US $6.5 million for operational research from 2009-2016.[2]

The first prevalence survey since the 1980s was completed by the International Center for Diarrheal Disease Research, Bangladesh in 2010, finally enabling policy-makers to access accurate information for strategy formulation. Further secondary analysis is planned and has the potential to further refine TB control efforts by pinpointing the most at risk populations. Mostafa Kamal at the National Institute of Diseases of the Chest and Hospital is currently leading a drug resistance surveillance study.

The Damien Foundation uses both Global Fund dollars and outside sources to conduct a range of research. Many of its research

---

[2] In the Round 8 Global Fund grant (2009-2013), USD $2 million was earmarked for operational research, and an additional USD $4.5 million was approved in Round 10 (2010-2015).

questions consider cost-benefit analysis for resource utilization in the Bangladesh context. For example, if the NTP changed its guidelines to conduct drug sensitivity testing on all patients that relapse after completing category one treatment, instead of first having them complete the Category II treatment regimen, how many additional MDR TB cases would it identify? What would be the additional burden on the laboratories, and would this have implications for the quality of their tests? Having in-country expertise to inform policy making greatly improves Bangladesh's ability to create policy that aligns with sound decisions about allocation of resources. Currently, the Damien Foundation is testing different regimens for MDR TB patients to see which regimens yield the best patient outcomes.[3]

5.4 Flexibility and evolution

As with any large-scale public health program, all partners must operate with some flexibility. As the partnership has matured, there are been some organic changes in responsibilities. For example, in the 1990s, all partnerships were initiated by the NTP. Since BRAC has become a principal recipient for the Global Fund, it has become much more involved in seeking out new partners, which it submits for approval to the NTP.

In relying on NGOs, the NTP recognizes that it has the ultimate responsibility for the quality standards of the program, and therefore it must be aware of potential consequences that NGO support can create. For example, one public sector official noted that NGO staff may receive intense pressure from their superiors to report high numbers. When the pressure is too intense, this can lead to inflation of the data. One NTP staff member describes, "as a government official, my position is protected, so I can be honest about our program performance. Using performance to motivate staff can be effective, but NGOs should be careful not to take it too far." While an NGO's ability to move quickly can be valuable, maintaining quality remains a parallel concern for all stakeholders.

---

[3] The result of one such study is: Deun AV, Maug AKJ, Salim MAH, PK Das, MR Sarker, P Daru, HL Reider (2010). Short, highly effective, and inexpensive standardized treatment of multi-drug resistant tuberculosis. *American Journal of Respiratory and Critical Care Medicine.* 82; 684-92.

5.5 Ongoing challenges for the NTP

Human resource challenges

The NTP faces significant human resource shortages. In 2010, only five out of 21 Global Fund-funded posts were filled (WHO, 2010, 46).While still significant, vacancies have decreased in recent years. For example, in 2005, more than half of all sub-districts had fewer than 80% of key staff positions filled. By 2010, only 20% still faced manpower shortages of this magnitude. One significant result of the staffing shortages was a reduced capacity to provide supervision. Central NTP staff also acknowledge their inability to spend as much time visiting programs as they'd like. BRAC at times must increase its staffing, particularly for laboratory services in hard-to-reach areas, to compensate for the public sector's shortages.

Bureaucracy

Lacking the broad mandate facing the Ministry of Health and Family Welfare, BRAC can organize its health program for its current needs. With the arrival of Global Fund resources, BRAC created a unit to manage its sub-contracts. These staff have a closer relationship with the financial office and therefore are able to ensure that payments occur as efficiently as possible.

As mentioned in Chapter 4, the WHO initially assumed responsibilities for holding the Global Fund resources dispersed to the NTP as it lacked the administrative capacity to manage them itself. In 2009, the Global Fund indicated that the WHO's participation in TB control did not facilitate country ownership and should be phased out. All funding allocated under the NTP's agreement funnels directly to the NTP, and the WHO receives 10% for the technical support that it provides. However, the NTP faces significant challenges in managing these funds, so while symbolically the phase out has occurred, the WHO continues to provide assistance to ensure that these administrative challenges do not compromise the program's operations.

Given the scope of responsibility facing the NTP, effective and sustained leadership is required. Many of the most urgent challenges will require significant investments and several iterations of improvements. System-level improvement in particular is inherently gradual and time intensive. Currently, the NTP program manager is not a fixed-term position, and length of tenure and qualifications can vary greatly. In the past few years, the NTP has experienced significant turnover in its leaders. This trend remains a challenge for the NTP and its partners in maximizing the current opportunity to create the best TB control system possible.

Infrastructure issues

Over the life of the Global Fund, all 460 sub-district health complexes have been equipped with a microscope. Nationwide, there are now approximately 1,000 laboratories engaged in the TB control program (Global Fund, 2009, 16/64). Though the basic infrastructure is now largely in place, ensuring quality remains problematic. Quality assurance for smear microscopy in most areas is sub optimal, and supervision by the national level is insufficient. Light emitting diode fluorescence microscopes are not used in most areas.

In addition, there is very limited ability to detect smear negative cases or extra-pulmonary TB. Most sub-district facilities lack x-ray machines and lack the expertise to diagnose extra-pulmonary TB or read an x-ray. Smear negative TB is a challenge to some of the chest disease clinics at well. In the cases where these services are available, they often cost the patient up to Tk 1,000 (US $14.30).

5.6 Creating a functional partnership

The partnership for TB control in Bangladesh has made huge strides since its birth in 1994. The prevalence survey completed in 2009, led by K. Zaman at the International Center for Diarrheal Disease Research, Bangladesh, found that the national adult prevalence rate of 79.4/100,000, a precipitous decline from the rate of 870/100,000 found in the 1987-1988 prevalence survey (ICDDRB, 2010). Nationwide, programs have intensified in service delivery and infrastructure; huge numbers of staff have been trained, new partnerships have been formed, and capacities to respond to new challenges in TB are being generated. However, in order to sustain its gains, members of the partnership are well aware that they must continue to push the program forward. While Global Fund funding is secured through 2016, there is no guarantee that these funds will be available indefinitely, so efforts must be aggressive and roll back the TB epidemic to a manageable level.

Some goals can be achieved through independent actors, but increasingly, there is value to collaboration and joint activity. Partners have different areas of expertise that can be leveraged more effectively, and epidemiological trends will require a full care delivery value chain of excellence—aggressive case findings, sophisticated diagnostic capabilities, and strong adherence support measures. By working together, partners can best control TB nationally. This requires investment in relationships, time for coordination and planning, and a system-level perspective.

Creating a partnership in a decentralized system

As discussed in Chapter 4, BRAC relies on its local offices to handle many situations on their own. It has invested significantly in building capacity within its leaders at the district and sub-district levels so that they have the skills, confidence, and sense of responsibility to respond effectively. Within this partnership model, relying on central support and decision-making inherently creates a lag time for responding. Creating local nodes of expertise and responsiveness will lead to faster and more efficient solutions to small-scale issues. Already, NGOs rely substantially on the clinical expertise of local sub-district health complexes and chest clinics. The current challenge is for sub-district and district level public sector staff to provide similar levels of supervisory support and monitoring. Joint monitoring is a powerful tool for institutionalizing a partnership and effectively motivating implementing partners to excel.

Public sector staff are told to organize meetings and conduct site visits, but no mechanisms exist from NTP to monitor whether these are completed regularly. Some NGOs have taken the initiative to strongly promote these meetings at the local level, sensing that getting buy-in from these leaders will inevitably strengthen TB control linkages and outcomes overall. For example, Damien Foundation field officers go to the government sub-district health complex on the day when all public field staff come to submit reports and collect their salary each month. They provide an update and feedback to these individuals, sharing any upcoming events or current challenges that need addressing. Through this more informal channel of relationship building, Damien Foundation is slowly building awareness and rapport with the field staff, who in turn demonstrate more commitment in fulfilling their activities within the scope of the TB control partner.

Maintaining relationships within the partnership

Often, public-private partnerships are characterized as NGOs against the government. While the NTP is the critical anchor of the program, relationships between NGOs range in intensity and character, creating instances of organic collaboration, absence of communication, or fierce competition, all of which have a significant impact on patient care. Erwin Cooremann, WHO, cautioned against seeing NGOs as one entity. "It's important to realize that they are individual institutions and they have important interactions within themselves. You can't expect them to always get along. These relationships are quite important to the effectiveness of the partnership."

Regular meetings are one way of building these institutional ties. Project proposal writing has been a catalyst for joint activity. Leveraging this opportunity to create more continuous coordination and planning will open the doors to another level of system improvement. A complicating factor to maintaining the strength of the partnership is the growing scale of the program that the additional funding has enabled. Khurshid Alam Hyder, WHO, reflects, "Those working on TB control used to be a close-knit group. I trained all the civil surgeons, *upazila* [sub-district] health and family planning officers, and medical officers of the country myself; I knew them all personally. As the program has grown, this is no longer the case." In addition, many of those who spent decades working on TB control have begun to retire or have moved internationally. After several years at the WHO, Khurshid recently became the Regional Adviser for the WHO Southeast Asia Regional Office, demonstrating that the opportunities to leverage Bangladesh's experience for other countries may mean that some individuals can no longer provide as much leadership locally. Salim, who led scale up of TB programming at the Damien Foundation, moved to KNCV Tuberculosis Foundation in the Netherlands. These individuals can facilitate regional partnerships and opportunities for international learning, but maintaining the quality of programming within Bangladesh requires ongoing cultivation of the next generation of leaders and relationships.

Leadership and sustainability

In 2010, the NTP supported the WHO in completing the fifth joint monitoring mission of the TB Control Program. The consultants included Marijke Becx, who had spent several years at the NTP in the early 2000s and assisted Bangladesh in developing its Global Fund proposals. Becx reflected that the initial intense focus on service delivery had enabled astonishing increases in the case detection and cure rates. As the backlog of cases decreases and the public sector service delivery capacity grows, the partnership is now well positioned to function as a joint entity. The NTP has ownership of the partnership and possesses this convening power, but may require the catalyzing push from the WHO or NGO partners to organize regular partnership-building activities. The absence of these creates potential for duplication and lack of coordination. NGOs can support the NTP if it provides the necessary guidance as to the direction in which all partners should be headed. One example of NGOs acting as a stopgap is BRAC's recruitment of new partners into the partnership. In some cases, BRAC signed a contract with these new partners prior to their finalization of with a memorandum of understanding the NTP to enable them to start delivering services more rapidly (WHO, 2010, 35).

Bangladesh's partnership is unique in the extent that NGOs provide service delivery. NGOs like BRAC and the Damien Foundation have demonstrated an ability to implement TB services on a large-scale and can greatly expand the NTP's reach. While NGOs are committed remaining in a supportive role and aim to contribute to public sector priorities, in the absence of sustained leadership from the NTP, walking this line can be challenging.

The government continues to reduce the amount of funding it contributes to TB control, though its indirect support, through the general health system budget and activities, remains strong. Currently, the Global Fund provides the vast majority of support for the program (Table 5.3).[4] As discussed, complete reliance on external funds creates institutional vulnerability if issues around funding arise. Commitment extends beyond the financial realm; the NTP and NGO partners also need to work together to keep TB on the national agenda. Ensuring sufficient political commitment for public funds

---

[4] Excludes salaries and infrastructure.

for the program if external sources wane is critical to long-term planning and success.

Table 5.3: National budget for TB control by source, 2009

Source	USD, millions
Government (excludes general health system expenditures)	0.432
World Bank	0.390
TB Control Assistance Program (USAID)	2.20
Global Fund	16.732
Total	**19.754**

Source: Bangladesh CCM, 2009, 50-51.

A selection of perspectives on the partnership

"Even then the partnership is going very well, this government becomes dependent on the partnership; anytime you go to the field to see the NGOs, they are doing well, but it's BRAC that's there supporting them, so ultimately they are dependent on them. This is not good for the sustainability of program, the government should take the ownership."
"All in all, the government had not taken leadership; sometimes they complained that the NGOs were too independent and doing too much but they didn't sit in the driver's seat."

"Successful partnership depends on attitude. This is the duty of the government to give health care services to the citizens. NGOs are supporting agencies, not parallel to the government. Must not think that they are parallel to government, that's when the problems arise. We are not facing this problem still today, but have to be careful to ensure that we prevent it happening in the future."

"We are happy with the progress that we are making with NGOs. We don't control funding for the government. I hope that they are seeing the effectiveness of the NGO part of the program. I hope that they learn from working with us and do their part to improve their functioning."

"The NTP needs to be in the driver seat. The NGOs are supposed to be helpers, sitting in the back, but if there is no driver, they might try to take over and steer."

In recent years, NGOs have tried to cultivate public awareness and support for TB control. In 2006, with support from the Open Society Institute, *Public Health Watch* developed a publication on civil society perspectives of TB policy in Bangladesh (Public Health Watch, 2006). It underscored the need for increased political commitment and leadership. George Soros came to Bangladesh to formally launch the report to raise the profile of the effort. In its recommendations, the publication encouraged greater advocacy efforts and visibility in the media. Garnering popular support for TB control is another lever to increase political commitment, which will become increasingly important as donors increasingly look for evidence of country ownership and sustainability in funding decisions.

5.7 Adapting the partnership

The Global Fund has radically altered the landscape for TB control in Bangladesh. Its grants have enabled Bangladesh to greatly intensify its service delivery and make critical improvements to its infrastructure. Now in its 7th year of implementing with Global Fund support, the NTP and its partners are poised to consider how to best utilize these new capacities for the current situation. Emerging data on multidrug resistant (MDR) TB trends and the recent prevalence survey provide guidance on the specific populations at risk.

As TB control evolves, the partnership becomes more critical to maintain. Creating mechanisms for partners to learn from each other will enable them to build on each other's strengths.

Current objectives of the partnership include: scale up of MDR TB diagnostic and treatment services, infection control, laboratory strengthening, procurement, community TB care, hard-to-reach areas and vulnerable groups, childhood TB, and DOTS expansion. Bangladesh is characterized by constant change, and any system to deliver treatment for chronic care must be durable. Investments by the government and external donors have enabled the public sector to increase its capacity significantly in recent years. Many of these expansions are synergistic: for example, the Ministry of Health and Family Welfare is upgrading 18,000 community health clinics to improve their capacity to provide antenatal care. It recognized that the investment that this would require, including hiring additional staff and improving facilities, would provide the infrastructure required for these sites to deliver DOTS services. These plans are approved and execution will begin in the summer of 2011. Clearly they will take time to implement fully as needed staff have to be recruited and trained. Nonetheless, NGOs should plan to gradually adjust their activities in response to better support these systemic improvements. As the public sector becomes better able to deliver basic services, NGOs need to work together to share lessons on how to tackle complex challenges. BRAC has much to learn from the Damien Foundation and other NGOs about controlling MDR TB and HIV-TB co-infection. By working together, partners can leverage each other's capacities and refine their own models. BRAC an offer lessons in community mobilization and managing at scale while it gains a deeper understanding of how to integrate needed forms of care into its existing model.

However, for the time being, the gains made in the public sector have yet to diminish the need for NGO contribution. "We've

> "The partnership needs strengthening in the sense of regular contact, and that's of increasing importance because TB control has become much complicated. BRAC in Round 3 and 5 did basic DOTS, but now there are more requirements, MDR TB, for instance, and the Damien Foundation has been providing related services for several years. BRAC could make much more use of NGOs that have technical expertise and capabilities in dealing with the more complex matters of TB control. All the NGOs will need to expand beyond just DOTS; they all need to be thinking about the more difficult fields HIV and TB, and MDR TB as well. They can't escape; they don't necessarily all need to do diagnosis; but they have to follow up cases, identify complications and side effects. In that respect, the partnership should also include sharing and monitoring and evaluation and experiences, by field visits."
>
> *Marijke Becx , formerly World Health Organization*

improved the health system infrastructure, but we're not expanding it fast enough to keep pace with the population growth," one government official commented. In addition to expanding basic program, there are specific populations and emerging epidemiological trends that require immediate responses to be contained. These include effective TB control in urban areas, co-infection between TB and HIV, and MDR TB.

Urban TB

As will be discussed in Chapter 7, urban TB control remains a national priority. One central challenge at the partnership level will be to devise an effective mechanism for engaging new partners into the partnership structures, particularly when they include private practitioners, industry partners and other non-traditional entities. Ongoing efforts in these areas are numerous, but uncoordinated. Efforts to create a national implementation strategy for engaging private providers are slow, and consequently intensity and types of follow up with individual providers varies between NGOs (WHO, 2010, 36).

Co-infection

Individuals with HIV and other immuno-compromising conditions experience an elevated risk for TB. In some contexts, TB can be an indication of undiagnosed HIV. Creating TB and HIV programs with linkages and active screening activities are examples of holistic program strategies. National level coordination enables these types of integration in guidelines and practice. Consequently, the NTP and the National AIDS and Sexually Transmitted Infections (STI) Program established a steering committee. As with the TB partnership itself, now that the groundwork has been established, the current challenge is creating a regular schedule of meetings and joint activities (WHO, 2010, 32).

In 2005, there were no active efforts to ensure that people living with HIV had access to TB screening and treatment. In 2010, over 50% of the estimated number of people co-infected with HIV and TB were receiving DOTS treatment for TB (NTP, 2006). In 2008 an NGO providing services to people living with HIV joined the partnership (See Chapter 7 for more details). The partnership has increasingly recruited new partners with experience in HIV to increase their ability to respond to the next generation of challenges in TB control. As NGOs interact through the partnership, they may be able to catalyze the national programs in their coordination and provide recommendations on how to tackle issues of co-infection.

MDR TB

While the available data is sparse, experts estimate that overall, Bangladesh has an MDR TB rate of 2.2% in new cases and 15.3% in re-treatment cases (5.5% overall) (WHO, 2011). The World Health Organization has named Bangladesh one of the 27 priority countries for controlling MDR and extensively drug resistant TB (XDR TB) (WHO, 2011).The Damien Foundation began treating MDR TB in its own facilities as early as 1997 and, based on its experience, it has been an advocate at the global level for a 9-month treatment course (vs. the current 24-month course recommended by the WHO). In 2006, the TB partnership began to discuss adding MDR TB to its priorities. In 2007, the National Institute of Diseases of the Chest and Hospital received funds to enroll 700 patients from the Global Fund (see table below for more details). However, preparing the facility and staff to treat MDR TB proved a greater challenge than the NTP had anticipated. Getting results on the drug sensitivity testing from the national reference laboratory alone took an average of three months. Finally, in 2008, the hospital began to enroll patients, and by June 2009, had enrolled just over 400 (BCCM, 2009, 11/64).

Table 5.4: Details on MDR TB programs in Bangladesh

	Damien Foundation	National Institute of Diseases of the Chest and Hospital (NIDCH)
Coverage area and population	Entire designated coverage area of 13 districts; recently expanded to cover all of Rajshahi division	Patients referred from all over the country except in DF-supported areas
Capacity	Three of its own facilities, also managing MDR treatment in Rajshahi Chest Hospital; reference lab with drug sensitivity testing (use rifampicin resistance as a surrogate for MDR TB)	NIDCH has 670 beds, 280 for TB and of those 130 beds designated for MDR-TB. Usually spillover to the non-MDR-TB ward due to the patient load.
Definition of suspect	Category 1 patient remaining positive at three months or more; Category 2 patients remaining positive at four months or more Relapses of both Cat 1 and 2, treatment after default Symptomatic contacts of MDR TB Patients	Category 2 patient remaining positive at 5 month, Category 2 patient remaining positive after 8 month, also under pilot (not currently national guidelines) Category 1 failure(remain positive at 6 month)
Regimen	Intensive Phase (4+ months):	Intensive Phase (6+ months):
	Kanamycin, Prothionamide Gatifloxacin, Pyrazinamide, Clofazimine, Ethambutol, Isoniazid	Pyrazinamide, Kanamycin (injection) Ofloxacin, Ethionamide, Cycloserine
	Continuation phase (5 months): Gatifloxacin, Pyrazinamide, Clofazimine, Ethambutol	Continuation Phase(18 + months): Pyrazinamide, Ofloxacin, Ethionamide, Cycloserine
Treatment details	TB/Leprosy control assistant and TB/Leprosy control officer informed of results. They trace, counsel, and refer patients to the hospital. Decision to treat made by the treating doctor.	DOTS-plus coordinator and team make treatment decisions. Monthly sputum culture and smear conducted DOTS not strictly adhered to for hospitalized patients; some adverse effects including GI system issues.

(contd.)

(Table 5.4 contd.)

	Damien Foundation	National Institute of Diseases of the Chest and Hospital (NIDCH)
	Treatment is a 4-7 month intensive phase followed by continuation phase of 5 months, which is overseen by the NGO partner working in the patient's home area. Culture sample conducted monthly during the intensive phase and at months 6, 8, and 9. Routine samples are collected every six months for two years following completion of treatment.	Policy for discharge is 4 negative cultures; earliest after 6 months, but usually at month 7-8. NTP prepares the DOT provider and provides the drug supply for ambulatory treatment.
Infection control measures	Wards are well-ventilated and provision of UV light at night or when doors and windows are closed. Patients wear cloth masks. Wards are fairly overcrowded. Infectious and drug resistant patients are segregated though share bathrooms and dining hall.	Some mixing of patients in wards, though wards are typically well ventilated and patients wear cloth masks.
Outcomes	In 2009: 164 patients were treated for MDR TB. 82% were cured, 10% defaulted, 6% died, 1% failed. In June 2011, 122 patients were under treatment.	643 culture-positive MDR TB patients diagnosed between August 2008-Sept 2010; 434 put on treatment; report on outcomes of first cohort to be released in fall 2011.
Cost per patient	US $312	US $2,345

Sources: WHO 2010, 25-30; pers. comm. with staff from Damien Foundation, University Research Company, LLC and National Institute of Diseases of the Chest and Hospital.

MDR TB control represents a significant increase in complexity to the basic DOTS structure that Bangladesh has scaled nationally. Country capacity to appropriately diagnose and support patients is crucial to minimizing the risk of XDR TB. Extensive planning for inflection control and avoidance of shortages of second-line medications cannot be overlooked. Bangladesh is proceeding cautiously and has delayed enrolling patients to ensure that its infrastructure is adequate before expanding too quickly. Technical capacity and program management both require additional investments to strengthen these activities. As a first case finding strategy, patients who fail the re-treatment regimen or test sputum positive at five months are assessed, and case management is based on hospitalization in the intensive phase. The NTP is currently reviewing the criteria for MDR TB suspects to test more broadly and assessing its capacity to treat the estimated increases in patients these revisions would yield.

The expanding MDR TB program underscores the importance of investing the partnership not just for symbolic reasons, but also for achieving good patient outcomes. The current protocol includes the passing of patients between providers; linkages and communication must be very strong to support this process and ensure that these patients maintain treatment through the transitions. Kamal Hossain, Damien Foundation, comments that, "At first it was difficult to ensure that we got the culture samples from the partners. There were a lot of administrative issues, and in many cases the NGOs were not really sure what to do. We'd have to call them to see if they were following up with the patient, and understand where the problem was. Now that we've taken the time to orient everyone and create written protocols for them to follow, it's rare that we don't get a culture back promptly." The Damien Foundation recognizes the joint responsibility that all partners in the area share in treating these patients, and is already convening regular meetings in the district to discuss MDR TB treatment plans. As MDR TB treatment scales up to new areas, such as Dhaka, not only will there be a need to expand technical and infrastructural capacity, but also the understanding and networks between partners to support patients from screening and diagnosis through vigilance after completing treatment.

Many second-line TB drugs are readily available in pharmacies at low prices. Failure to strengthen the regulatory environment will threaten the effectiveness of any MDR TB effort, as these drugs are being dispersed freely without the mechanisms of adherence support, drug sensitivity testing, and physician supervision that reduce the risks of furthering drug resistance. NGO partners can advocate for these changes, but ultimately these policy level changes rest on political commitment and action.

5.8 Conclusions

Public-private partnerships are full of challenges, frustrations, and energy-intensive activities, and require intense investments. Despite these downsides, they represent one of the best strategies for improving health in countries like Bangladesh, where a mosaic of partners can provide pockets of capabilities that are harnessed to contribute to a larger system. The TB partnership in Bangladesh provides many lessons to other countries attempting to use the partnership model for its own disease control efforts. While its gaps and weaknesses are of note, its results offer compelling evidence that the strategy has great potential. We demonstrate the potential reflections for others based on our experience in Bangladesh:

There is no substitute for government leadership. Partnerships require a leader to provide a vision, guidelines, enforcement, and ongoing support. Government departments are not always set up with structures and policies that are conducive to these roles. Nonetheless, the public sector is the only entity with the legitimacy to provide this role, and its absence will inevitably hurt the partnership. Others, such as NGOs, can support the government in some of the responsibilities, but the public sector must take and exercise its leadership continuously.

Partnerships require active management and institutionalization. Every good manager knows that to keep his team running smoothly, he must invest time in management activities and systems. Similarly, a partnership must be proactively managed. Often coordination activities get postponed or canceled in the urgency of implementation challenges, but they are crucial for maintaining quality over time. While strong relationships between partners enable constant informal lines of communications, planned activities allow leaders to establish a shared vision, facilitate cross-partner learning, and codify the partnership itself, allowing it to sustain beyond the term of the individual partners or leaders. Smaller meetings allow stakeholders to focus on technical issues with more efficiency, but also will be insufficient without the larger strategic picture being communicated to all.

Partners must internally promote the partnership approach and build capacity. While regular meetings and coordination are essential, without active buy-in from partners, they will not yield optimal results. Leadership must encourage transparency, the sharing of successes and failures, and a genuine desire for other partners to thrive. Sharing successful innovations is important, but equally as significant is sharing a challenge or performance data that one would prefer to hide. Metrics such as the return rate of referrals speak of the strength of partnership, but less quantifiable signs, such as the frequency of informal communication or creation of opportunities for learning exchanges, can also be indicative.

Infrastructure requires significant support and supervision. In the past seven years, Bangladesh has greatly expanded its laboratory capacities nationally. It has built a number of new labs, created the capability for drug sensitivity testing, and implemented an external quality assurance program. However, these systems require support and supervision to ensure their functioning and proper usage. Service delivery hinges on strong diagnostic abilities; otherwise treatment will be inefficient and potentially spur drug resistance. Supervision, particularly when conducted comprehensively, enables rapid identification and discussion of weaknesses and instills accountability among all partners for their practices and results. External mechanisms, such as quality assurance measures for laboratories, confirm technical quality of services, so long as they are properly supervised and monitored on their practices. When funds are tight, often infrastructure suffers, as data on patients treated and cured is usually the focus nationally and for donors. Infrastructural investments are required for sustained success, and while less visible, are vital for TB control. Partnerships should advocate for sufficient funding for the necessary infrastructural components and protect dedicated resources for these purposes.

Effective TB control requires constant updating. One of the greatest advantages of a partnership approach is that it creates a "deep bench," that is, a team of diverse players can be assembled to best tackle the current epidemiological context. The TB control partnership in Bangladesh represents a range of expertise—from the sophisticated clinical activities to reaching individuals with HIV and TB to providing community-based DOTS support in hard-to-reach areas. No partner can simultaneously excel in all activities, but as a group, they can draw on all these capabilities. As the epidemic inevitably changes, partners must be vigilant in refining their strategy. New partners in professional associations, the private sector and other industries may be required; new populations, such as children, may represent segments that should be aggressively targeted. New technologies should be evaluated on whether they are appropriate for Bangladesh. Partnerships enable a range of expertise to be constantly assembled to discuss these issues together. With the mechanisms to facilitate these dialogs and then translate them into practice, partnerships can enable countries like Bangladesh to tackle TB.

Chapter 6

The Last Mile: Community Health Workers and Their Patients

6.1 Introduction

Community health workers and volunteers are a crucial response strategy to the shortages of human resources for health worldwide. Though now widely accepted as a valuable workforce, early pioneers of this approach faced significant skepticism and resistance from the medical community. However, in places like flood-prone Sulla, home to BRAC's earliest health programs, it was evident that models reliant exclusively on facilities or scarce physicians were inadequate to address all the community's health needs.

In the simplest terms, the driving philosophy behind BRAC's programs was "taking health to the people," which led them to the idea that village women could be the first line of public health service and limited curative care. Each volunteer provides value to their community, which BRAC anticipated meant that there was an opportunity for this role to generate income for her. BRAC has spent decades refining its model to create mechanisms of accountability and responsiveness so that *shebikas* are best prepared and motivated to meet the health needs of their community. These are not specific to BRAC's TB control activities, but are an important strength of its model. Similarly, while the majority of this book focuses on the specifics of the *shebika*'s role in TB control, these tasks are only a small component of her overall workload. The larger context is important for understanding *shebika* effectiveness and capabilities. In addition, the more recent addition of another layer of community health workers, called *shasthya kormis* (health worker), demonstrates that task shifting at the community level can require simultaneous and coordinated deployment of multiple types of lay health workers. BRAC's programmatic experiences are instructive in considering the critical areas to consider in designing, scaling, and managing a large cadre of community health workers.

6.2 A brief background on community health workers

Several studies have shown that community health workers are an effective, low-cost strategy for delivery of primary health care (Standing and Chowdhury, 2008). The likelihood of the community health worker delivering value varies on the model. Some of the determinants include: the selection of tasks, availability of appropriate supplies and equipment, coverage and equity, and cost of delivering services (relative to other models) (Berman, Gwatkin and Burger, 1985). Researchers have noted that in addition to performing health activities, community health workers offer more intangible benefits as well: they are likely to be socially embedded in communities in a stable and long-lasting way, and as a result, gain trust and confidence of individuals. They are well positioned to understand and empathize with patients. In many cases, community health workers are female and may be predisposed to serving women, particularly important in contexts where women's access to health services is limited (Standing and Chowdhury, 2008). These considerations suggest that the use of a community-based health cadre could also have longer-term influences on community mobilization, behaviors, and norms, if the program is maintained over time (Berman, Gwatkin and Burger, 1985).

Despite the clear potential value of community health workers, examples of failed programs abound. Explanations for these program outcomes usually fall into two categories. The first is economic and structural factors, usually related to government policy and waning support for the program in the midst of recessions or budgetary challenges. The second is the ambiguity about regulation, appropriate payment, and concerns about quality assurance that can also lead to controversy and disbandment of community health worker programs (Berman, Gwatkin and Burger, 1985).

6.3 Community-based health delivery in Bangladesh: The value proposition

In Bangladesh, a health system that relies on fixed site care delivery will be highly inaccessible to rural and poor communities for some time. Informal care providers offer more proximate options, but these lack any form of regulation or quality control.

While proximity could appeal to all villagers, those with limited means of transport and mobility would benefit the most from a local option, as no other options were within their reach. Door-to-door activities combated the prevailing norm of not seeking care until the crisis point was reached. In addition, they also create an opportunity for preventative screenings and care.

> "CHWs [community health workers] must be adequately supported and that such adequate support requires more resources than are now spent on CHW programs. CHWs cannot be seen as a marginal addition to existing services, funded by limited one-time special expenditures. If they are to have a significant impact, they must be an integral and effective component of the health system, and they must be funded as such...under-funding CHWs will merely extend inadequate services."
>
> *Berman et al., 1985*

A female cadre of community-based health workers creates access for women, who may lack the necessary support from their husband or mother-in-law to seek medical services. In addition to their having limited access to cash, women often were unable or unwilling to seek care from a male provider. Both in government clinics and in private options, almost all formal providers are traditionally male.

Shebikas also have the ability to improve health at the community level, in addition to the value that they offer individual patients. Many of the activities that BRAC expects from them, including surveillance, active case finding, health education, and distribution of preventive and curative goods, reduce incidence and transmission of disease, resulting in indirect health improvements for whole community.

BRAC's *shebika* model grew directly out of the village organization. The first *shebikas* were volunteers that primarily served the health needs of the other members of the group. Over time, the population and needs served by the *shebika* have expanded. Choosing additional services and products requires BRAC to maintain a deep knowledge of community and individual health needs.

6.4 Community and patient characteristics

BRAC has chosen to focus on the poor and marginalized; in Bangladesh, nearly 30% of the total population lives on under US $1 a day (BBS, 2011). Who are they? Though there has been substantial urban migration since independence, Bangladeshis are primarily rural dwellers, and subsistence farming is common. A large number rely primarily on their own harvest to sustain their family. An illness like tuberculosis can threaten the fragile grasp on survival. In the cases where the breadwinner dies, the family may have long-term economic hardships. Women have limited freedoms compared to men and are significantly underrepresented in the formal economy, creating high levels of dependence on men to provide for their household.

Strategic choices for health delivery: providing low-cost health services to the maximum number of people

Select specific types of patient problems. Matching the needs of patients with the capabilities of the organization. BRAC minimizes input variation by keeping the list of health conditions it treats directly (vs. referring) relatively short.

Select the right people and skill sets. The more highly trained staff an organization selects, the more complexity and variation of conditions they can address. Drawing on the pool of rural women who have few formal opportunities in the formal economy, BRAC creates a cadre of community health workers with few technical abilities, limiting for what conditions and level of variability its program can manage. These women work on a volunteer or honorarium basis and therefore are much less costly than highly trained medical professionals.

Use "appropriate" resources and technologies. BRAC keeps a lean inventory of resources and technology, though recently some of its programs have begun to pilot the use of mobile phones in health delivery. While they are unable to diagnose complex cases, these limitations allow them to keep capital costs low.

Framework drawn from: Bohmer, 2010

As discussed in Chapter 2, even in the 1970s, BRAC saw that a certain portion of the illness in villages could be prevented or treated by simple health products or behavioral changes. Barriers fell into three main categories: inability to pay, difficulty of access, and inaction. The third is perhaps the least obvious: most rural dwellers tended to treat illness themselves and not visit a health provider. In the late 1980s, BRAC found that only 10% of rural dwellers sought formal medical care when they were sick (Amin et al., 1989). In the cases that people choose to seek treatment, non-qualified village doctors or pharmacies were usually the most proximate options.

The shebika's customers

Not all villagers will choose to seek services from a community health volunteer with limited training. But as the *shebika* does not receive a fixed salary from BRAC, she's reliant on the community for compensation. In order to be most effective, she will need to identify those villagers with needs that align with her services and products, and she needs to market to them effectively. Additional factors such as her ability to build relationships to create a base of repeat customers, convince villagers to buy from her rather than other sources, and have opportunities to explain the importance of various products will also impact her sales ability. Indeed, a BRAC research study found that over 90% of all sales were made by repeat customers (Reichenbach and Shimul, in press).[1]

Members of the village organization make up almost half of the customer share. Mothers often buy medications for their children. Overall, women are the primary buyers, representing about 75% of sales. However, for some specific services, such as TB control, men are the main consumers. Three quarters of the *shebika*'s patients are extremely poor.

In one sense, these data indicate that BRAC has correctly identified the needs of a specific segment of the population and matched the *shebika*'s basket of goods accordingly. High levels of repeat customers indicate that there are high levels of satisfaction with the quality of services and goods. However, as many of BRAC's

---

[1] The objective of this study was to evaluate the financial sustainability of the shebika model for shebikas and for BRAC, and its transferability to other settings. In Bangladesh, researchers interviewed 270 *shebikas* in 30 sub-districts. Sub-districts with malaria and/or maternal, neonatal, and child health programs were excluded, as the focus was on the essential health care program.

shebikas now operate in areas without microfinance, their sales may suffer without the built in pool of customers that it offers. In addition, her income is coming from a small fraction of the community; capturing more "market share" would increase her profits.

What would this require? Improved skills? More products? Better integration with BRAC's other programs? Who are the customers, and what are their needs? Defining the market enables BRAC to design a strategy to continue to increase value that *shebikas* offer to their communities and their ability to benefit through their health-related activities.

6.5 Evolution of BRAC's model: *Shasthya shebikas* and *shasthya kormis*

> "When we started, villages were so isolated. Very few had vehicles and travel was difficult. There were not even pharmacies in most places. If people got sick, they had nowhere to go. We thought, if we could just create a system so that in the village, there was someone with a little bit of health knowledge and a few supplies, and who could give them a referral, that would be a big improvement."
>
> *Jalaluddin Ahmed, BRAC*

The environment in which BRAC's TB control program began was barren compared to what exists today. As a result, the *shebika*'s evolving role adaptations to the *shebika* model illustrate how a durable program can continually evolve to deliver value, despite numerous contextual changes. Failure to adequately appreciate the context has led to moments of high turnover or compromising of quality. Designing and managing the program in a way that allows for it to evolve dynamically is central to long-term effectiveness. In addition, while functions and major activities can and should change periodically, core systems should be sustained. A strong supply chain, good supervision, monitoring, linkages and partnerships are a few key capabilities that all delivery systems require to perform optimally. As BRAC scaled its TB program beyond the reach of the microfinance program, BRAC thought that additional supervision would be one way to compensate and ensure quality of treatment. Furthermore, if supervision also came from the villages and was provided by a woman with more education, she could simultaneously increase the number of services provided at the community level. In 2003, BRAC Afghanistan created a new cadre of health workers as a response to the geographic challenges, and BRAC decided to introduce the *shasthya kormi* (health worker) role in the Bangladesh context as well (see Chapter 8 for more information on BRAC's program in Afghanistan). These health workers would not replace the *shebikas*, but complement and enhance their work.

6.6 *Shasthya shebikas*

Since its pilots in the 1970s, BRAC's *shasthya shebika* has evolved into what BRAC now calls the essential health care program and has scaled dramatically, both in terms of the scope of activities and geographic coverage (Figure 6.1). Currently, BRAC supervises over 89,000 *shebikas* in Bangladesh, which covered a population of over 110 million in 2010. *Shebikas* provide a range of health services and continue to express a desire to expand into still further areas. In the past ten years, BRAC has also expanded in urban areas, stretching the model in new ways.

Figure 6.1: Number of active *shebikas* in Bangladesh, 2003-2011

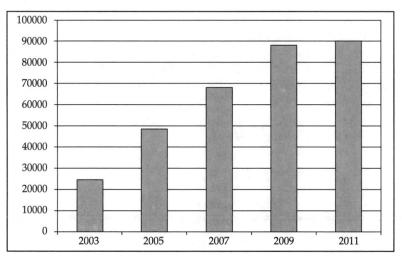

Criteria and selection

Over time, BRAC has learned a great deal about the selection of women to be effective *shebikas*. Having experienced the impact of high level of turnover, they've developed precise criteria for the position. Typically, one becomes a *shebika* after nominating oneself or being approached by the program organizer. Rarely does the *shasthya kormi* play a role in the process; her involvement begins once the selection process has concluded. The village organization must approve the *shebika* in order for her to begin training. Local government health staff are informed and can participate in the process if they desire. Usually a *shebika* is selected within 1-2 months of starting the search.

For many years, membership in the village organizations was required for *shebikas*. During the 1990s, when the tuberculosis program expanded beyond the range of microfinance programming, *shebikas* were given the option of joining the new village organizations or terminating their role. In the 2000s, as the health program grew still more with the influx of Global Fund resources, BRAC dropped this criterion in recognition that these programs were no longer as tightly bound as they had been in their early days. Currently, in communities with a village organization, BRAC will begin its search for a *shebika* by soliciting volunteers from the members. If a suitable candidate with required characteristics cannot be found, women outside of the village organization will be considered, though BRAC will encourage them to join to be incorporated more fully into BRAC's activities and gain access to microfinance.

Current criteria for a *shebika*:

- She is married and her youngest child is not less than two years of age
- She is 25 years or older
- She is willing to provide voluntary services
- She is socially acceptable to the village
- Her family agrees to her involvement
- She has five years or more of schooling

These criteria were developed based on a combination of observations in the field about which characteristics high-performing *shebikas* shared along with formal research from RED on what factors correlated with dropout. Women usually move to their husband's village after marriage, so married women are less likely to relocate. Young children generally require a lot of their mothers' time, and BRAC finds that *shebikas* often are not able to balance the dual sets of responsibilities for long. Family approval is also an important factor in turnover, so program organizers often spoke with a shebika's family as part of the selection process. In addition, acceptance from the major social structures surrounding her—family, village organization, and local elites—is central to her effectiveness and ability to generate sales. As the role does not include a salary, it is critical that she have the social capital to generate demand and inspire trust.

During the early years, *shebikas* were largely illiterate due to the relative lack of primary education available, particularly for women. Educational attainment has increased nationally, and BRAC is now able to require five years of schooling for *shebikas*. As *shebikas* are the primary collectors of data at the village level, their literacy enables them to better understand the health needs of communities. However, the increasing educational attainment levels mean that women serving as *shebikas* may have higher opportunity costs, motivating them to demand more from BRAC. These issues will be discussed in more depth below.

Characteristics of current shebikas

Women usually become *shebikas* in their early 30s (Rahman and Tasneem, 2008, 4).[2] Most have some schooling but only very basic literacy (Table 6.1). About 40% of current *shebikas* were village organization members at the time of their selection (Reichenbach and Shimul, in press). An additional 30% had been village organization members when selected and had since ceased to participate in the group. Some *shebikas* see membership in the village organization as a way to increase community trust in her role, resulting in higher demand and sales. Other RED studies show a higher proportion of *shebikas* in the village organizations (73%), with about a third

---

[2] Rahman and Tasneem's study explored changes in income earning capability in new and old *shebikas* due to the introduction of maternal, neonatal, and child health activities in a northern district of Bangladesh. It surveyed a randomly drawing sample of 764 *shebikas*, of which 453 were new and 311 were experienced.

becoming members only once they've begun to work as a *shebika* (Rahman and Tasneem, 2008, 5).

Table 6.1: Socio-demographic characteristics of current *shebikas*

Indicator	Average
Age	39 years
Number of years of schooling	5
Number of family members	5
Currently a village organization member	41%

BRAC has invested a few studies to better understand the financial situation of rural *shebikas*. A recent report found that most *shebikas* had other sources of livelihood in addition to their work as a *shebika*. Three quarters had or were raising poultry, which provided them with about Tk 300 (US $4) a month (Reichenbach and Shimul, in press). Handicraft work was another common activity (26%), providing about Tk 600 (US $8) a month.

However, there appears to be significant regional variation in *shebika* engagement in other forms of livelihood. A 2008 study focused on six sub-districts in the northeastern district of Nilphamari found that 61% of *shebikas* have no other income generating activities and 13% are engaged in agricultural work (Rahman and Tasneem, 2008, 7). Informal interviews in urban areas found that *shebikas* felt that their responsibilities for BRAC left little time for other employment.

Responsibilities

Each *shebika* is responsible for one village or approximately 200-250 households. *Shebikas* are expected to spend four hours working per day, six days per week, and conduct an average of 10-30 house visits daily. Survey data shows that women tended to spend about 3.5 hours a day working. Once *shebikas* are established in the community, people will seek out their services and products, thus expanding from the initial household-visit model. Most *shebikas* do not view their work as interfering with their ability to complete their duties at home (Reichenbach and Shimul, in press). A *shebika* serves primarily as a salesperson of health commodities; on average she has 30 transactions a month (see Table 6.2 for list of activities). With regards to TB treatment, *shebikas* usually have two patients under treatment at any given time.

Increasingly, *shebikas* are also incorporated into government community-based programming. The community health workers employed in the public sector cover a much larger catchment area than BRAC's *shebikas*, so they lack the intimate knowledge that these women acquire. Therefore, when they have a targeted intervention to conduct, for example, distribution of vitamin capsules to children under five, they can be more efficient by tapping into the *shebika*'s knowledge of which households contain members of their target population. *Shebikas* rarely provide service delivery for government programs (with TB control as the major exception), but routinely provide support and mobilization. These activities are not compensated by BRAC or the Ministry of Health and Family Welfare.

Table 6.2: *Shebika* **scope of work**

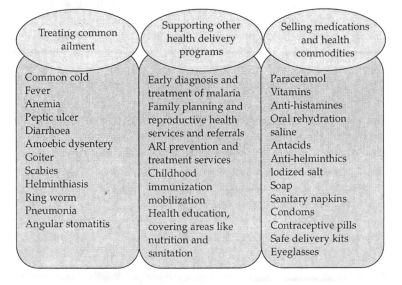

Treating common ailment	Supporting other health delivery programs	Selling medications and health commodities
Common cold	Early diagnosis and	Paracetamol
Fever	treatment of malaria	Vitamins
Anemia	Family planning and	Anti-histamines
Peptic ulcer	reproductive health	Oral rehydration
Diarrhoea	services and referrals	saline
Amoebic dysentery	ARI prevention and	Antacids
Goiter	treatment services	Anti-helminthics
Scabies	Childhood	Iodized salt
Helminthiasis	immunization	Soap
Ring worm	mobilization	Sanitary napkins
Pneumonia	Health education,	Condoms
Angular stomatitis	covering areas like	Contraceptive pills
	nutrition and	Safe delivery kits
	sanitation	Eyeglasses

Training

Once selected, all new *shebikas* receive a 15-day basic orientation training at the BRAC regional area office. Additional trainings are held on the more complex health conditions. For example, *shebikas* who will be performing TB control activities attend an additional 3-day training.

Shebikas are expected to attend monthly refresher trainings in their sub-district with the program organizer and *shasthya kormis*. At these trainings, *shebikas* and *shasthya kormis* share problems that they've experienced and observed in the field. For example, a *shebika* worries that when she falls sick, she may be unable to follow up on her TB patients if they fail to come to her house for treatment. Or, if many women in the community are asking how to increase their production at breast milk, the training is an opportunity to push that question to those with more training and get an answer to take back to one's community. In addition, the training is also an opportunity for *shebikas* to learn about new health initiatives or emerging issues. *Shebikas* also make work plans for the following month, including any campaigns or educational activities in their village.

Snapshot of the program organizer
Criteria: Twelve years of schooling
Length of initial training once selected: 12-day course; occasional additional trainings
Hours of work: Full-time
Primary activities: Supervise *shasthya kormi* and *shasthya shebikas*; conduct refresher trainings; replenish *shebika* health product inventory; collect data from the field level; and perform other administrative duties

While these trainings provide an important platform for continual maintenance of *shebika* skills, BRAC feels that one of its important functions is that it allows the *shebikas* to work as a team and enjoy a sense of collegiality with one another. Group problem-solving is both a form of support and opportunity to share discoveries and prevents the sense of isolation or being overwhelmed that can plague community-based volunteers.

Supervision

It has been noted in academic literature that performance-based financing models often require higher levels of supervision in order to avoid distortions in activity (Elridge and Palmer, 2009). *Shebikas* have two direct supervisors: a program organizer and a *shasthya kormi*, both of whom receive compensation from BRAC.

Program organizers supervise both the *shasthya kormi* and her *shasthya shebikas*. For both, he or she provides administrative and logistical support; these activities include organizing refresher trainings, providing health products, and overseeing payment for the TB program and other incentive-based programs. While the most of direct supervision for the *shebikas* comes from the *shasthya kormi*, the program organizer also provides technical support for some of the health programs. For example, he or she is responsible for monitoring the sputum collection process of the TB program.

Costs

The cost to BRAC for a *shebika* in her first year of service is about Tk 6,263 (US $90) and Tk 2,393 (US $34) in subsequent years (Reichenbach and Shimul, in press). Trainings and supervision are the major expenses. An additional factor in the higher costs for the first year is BRAC's responsiveness to the time required for a new *shebika* to gain recognition from the community. Government field staff must also be informed and usually reminded of her identity a few times before they begin to seek her out directly when they visit her village for public programs. BRAC staff estimate that more intense support is required for the first 5-7 months and then tapers to the routine schedule.

Clearly, *shebika* turnover is expensive for BRAC, and retention strategies are important in keeping costs manageable. Furthermore, over time, a *shebika* gains technical skills, trust of her community, and relationships with government staff in her area over time, so her value grows. Retention of *shebikas* has been a particular issue in urban areas (this is discussed in Chapter 7), and BRAC notes the difficulty in maintaining programs without a consistent cadre at the front line.

Competition

Shebikas are largely motivated by opportunities to make money. With the expansion of the public and private health sector, the goods that the *shebika* provides are now also available from nearby pharmacies. Most also face competition from unqualified doctors (also known as "quacks" or "village doctors"), and in some cases government facilities create competition as well (Reichenbach and Shimul, in press).

As in other industries, brand and customer preferences are important determinants of the *shebika*'s success. Her ability to differentiate herself from the competition is an important contributor to her ability to make sales. Negative perceptions of public facilities may lead customers to seek her services instead. BRAC's medicines also come professionally wrapped, unlike the loose pills that public dispensaries and some pharmacies provide, allowing for easier storage and reducing the risk of contamination. Through house visits and in some cases, availability by mobile phone, *shebikas* often try to compete on the basis of convenience. They've also invested in relationship building to establish a base of loyal customers.

6.7 Income and other benefits

A *shebika's* total income will be the profit she receives from selling health products and providing services for which either customers or BRAC pay. For example, BRAC compensates her Tk 150 (US $2.15) for the six months of daily support she provides to each TB patient who completes the full course of treatment. BRAC pays *shebikas* Tk 20 for every pregnancy they identify and Tk 30 for connecting a pregnant woman with a *shasthya kormi* for prenatal care. In some catchment areas, *shebikas* receive a payment for certain referrals to health care facilities (Rahman and Tasneem, 2008, 13). When a household installs a slab latrine or a tube-well, she receives 10% of the cost from BRAC.

Can a *shebika* do that?[3]

As BRAC surveys other health conditions that *shebikas* could address at the community level, it must analyze:

- What is the nature of the medical condition? (What are the symptoms? How is it diagnosed?)

- What is the nature of the treatment? (How much variation exists in treatment outcomes? how much clinical judgment is required?)

- How well is the condition understood? What tools exist for prevention, diagnosis, and treatment/management?

These questions help determine whether the BRAC has the capabilities to effectively respond to a health issue. The answers to these questions change due to scientific advancements and breakthroughs in clinical medicine. Over time, knowledge about a given medical condition becomes increasingly codified, and health delivery can be further protocolized and less reliant on the clinical expertise of an individual physician.

After accounting for recovering the costs of the medications that the *shebika* pays BRAC, she makes on average Tk 375 (US $5.50) per month. Income usually increases over time, with new *shebikas*

---
[3] Framework drawn from: Bohmer, 2010.

averaging Tk 275 (US $3.93) per month (Reichenbach and Shimul, in press).[4] While these amounts may seem relatively low, most *shebikas* see them as having a substantial impact on household income. *Shebikas* often use the money on their children or to purchase food for the household, though some are able to put it into savings (Reichenbach and Shimul, in press).

Shebikas benefit in non-monetary dimensions as well, often gaining importance at the family level and social acceptability more broadly (Ahmed, 2009). Their access to informal credit markets improves, and almost all note an increase in their financial independence (Reichenbach and Shimul, in press). Almost half report improvements in their own health status. In general they perceive many additional social improvements as a result of their work, including importance at family level and social acceptability (Rahman and Tasneem, 2008, 32-33). One *shebika* interviewed said, "If I worked in other households, I could earn a fixed amount of money but all the villagers would not have called me 'BRAC doctor.' For this I am working as a SS (*shasthya shebika*) (Ahmed, 2010)." When BRAC has conducted satisfaction surveys, *shebikas* generally indicate high levels of contentment with the nature of the work, as it allows them to work from home, enjoy relatively good hours, and gain social prestige (Reichenbach and Shimul, in press). Having outside training was significantly associated with serving a longer term of service as a *shebika* (Rahman and Tasneem, 18).

In the late 1990s, BRAC's research and evaluation division undertook a study of *shebika* dropout and found an annual dropout rate of 3.2%, relatively low compared to rates reported by other programs with health volunteers (Standing and Chowdhury, 2008). The major motivation for dropout included:

- Financial compensation inadequate for the time required,
- Time constraints from household chores,
- Disapproval from husband and other family members,
- Criticism from neighbors on religious grounds, and
- People's unwillingness to pay for services; skepticism of *shebika* legitimacy as provider.

---

[4] This study excluded income from TB treatment, so total monthly income will be higher for *shebikas* providing DOTS.

Thirteen percent of current *shebikas* surveyed had considered dropping out, with four out of five of these women unhappy with what they saw as a low level of compensation for their work. Despite the impact that current income levels provide, the demand for reasonable, fixed monthly salary is a "recurrent theme" of BRAC's internal and external assessments of the program (Ahmed, 2010). While BRAC has no plans to introduce a fixed salary based primarily on concerns about sustainability, discussions and experiments to provide additional incentives and opportunities for compensations are ongoing. Surveys from the field investigating the potential to create new, non-monetary incentives found that some *shebikas* would be interested in receiving an umbrella (33%) and a trunk (8%) for their activities (Rahman and Tasneem, 2008, 29).

6.8 *Shebika* performance

Shebika performance appears to be driven not by quantity of activities, but choices of activities and resources. Many high performers received training from outside of BRAC, such as midwifery (Rahman and Tasneem, 2008, 17). They tend to be village organization members and take a loan from BRAC. Perhaps due to their relatively high level of sales, virtually all replenish their supplies between refresher trainings, and compared to lower performers, they tend to buy a wide variety of products from BRAC and are more likely to stock their basket with outside supplies (Reichenbach and Shimul, in press).

A *shebika*'s income is influenced by many individual factors, such as her experience and interpersonal communication skills. The social capital that she develops over time, as she builds a reputation and gains community acceptability, increases her income. As mentioned, competition or remoteness also has an impact on income, with BRAC's analyses showing that in areas that lack access to public services, *shebikas* tend to have higher income levels.

6.9 Updating the *shebika* model: Trade-offs

"In the eighties and the nineties, when the EHC/SS [essential healthcare/ *shasthya shebika*] model was being developed, the scenario in the rural areas was quite different compared to the beginning of the 21st century. In the '80s, the economy was only beginning to gain momentum after the fall out of war and natural disasters, and the mobility and opportunities for the rural women were limited. Besides involvement in the family planning program of the government, large-scale employment of women in income-earning activities at the grassroots level was virtually absent. To work as a community health provider and earn a modest sum of money was quite rewarding for the rural women at that time besides social recognition, prestige etc. However, the scenario has changed over time and income-earning opportunities have increased for rural women in different sectors (ready-made garment, poultry, non-agricultural activities sponsored by the NGOs etc.). The opportunity cost of being involved in low-return activity like SS's, has also increased. So, how can we maintain her motivation and retention in an era of increasing opportunities for rural women?"

Ahmed, 2010

In 2009, BRAC held a meeting to discuss the essential health care program and consider different strategies for updating the *shebika* model. The workshop revealed that considering the premise on which the *shebika* model is built is crucial in determining potential strategies for improvement. For example, BRAC had deliberately chosen a member of the village organization to be a *shebika* as a visible way for a poor, marginalized woman to deliver value to the community. She was able to access poor women easily, and with time, the local elite also accepted her services and products. However, with the current literacy rates, many at BRAC think that it's time to create higher criteria for the *shebikas*. This likely would mean that they don't belong to poorest segment of the society, but they could be taught to perform more complex forms of care, such as blood pressure monitoring and management of hypertension (Rohde and Buiya, 2010). Similarly, increasing compensation might entice women with more ability and improve retention rates, but it might reduce the number of *shebikas* that are from BRAC's target groups. BRAC must decide is this is a reasonable trade-off for increasing availability and potentially quality of services available at the community level.

Shebikas themselves recognize that they must be able to fulfill a basic level of their community's health needs to maintain its respect and trust. For example, first aid is an emergent need that they are not equipped to handle, despite community expectations that they provide services in these situations (Ahmed, 2010). But the more services that go into the *shebikas* basket, the more time she needs to work if she is not to neglect some of her duties. These are not easy issues to predict or even necessarily monitor, so BRAC is starting small in initiatives to introduce redesigns.

One pilot is testing the concept of a "model *shebika*." In 2010, BRAC selected 35 women in Dhaka that in addition to meeting the *shebika* criteria were literate and owned grocery stores. They agreed to not only conduct household visits, but also to supply their stores with BRAC health products, providing consumers a fixed place to come for goods and services. In return, BRAC provides them with access to a revolving fund of Tk 2,000 (US $27). While the pilot is still ongoing, preliminary evaluations demonstrate that the selection criteria were relaxed in a few cases, creating difficulty in interpreting the results and raising questions about the feasibility of the model. Despite these challenges, it appears that the model *shebikas* have achieved high levels of visibility in their communities, and many consumers seek them out at their shops. However, the model *shebikas* often split duties of manning the store with a husband or other family members and are not always present when a customer arrives. They also report difficulty in balancing household visits with the stores' needs, though they still request additional training. Many are already indicating that the revolving fund, while helpful in purchasing supplies, is inadequate for their efforts and are requesting a fixed salary or increased monetary incentives (Khan and Ahmed, 2011).

6.10 *Shasthya kormis*

As mentioned, the original impetus for the *shasthya kormi* arose in Afghanistan, as a difficult terrain made it challenging for program organizers to provide sufficient support to *shebikas* on their own. *Shasthya kormis* enabled program organizers to supervise more *shebikas* without compromising their access to support in the field. The model was brought back to Bangladesh with the idea that it could both reduce costs and bolster the capacity for service delivery in the communities. In 2011, there were over 7,900 *shasthya kormis* in BRAC's program (see Figure 6.2).

Most *shasthya kormis* participated in BRAC's programs as *shebikas* or other BRAC programs prior to joining in their current position (Zahan, 2010). Promising *shasthya kormi* candidates are usually identified by the PO and then recommended for an interview with the sub-district manager. The hiring process can also include a visit to the candidate's house to speak with her husband and ensure his support for her employment. *Shasthya kormis* also take a written exam at BRAC's sub-district office to test their proficiency in a range of

Figure 6.2: Number of active *shasthya kormis* in Bangladesh, 2003-2011

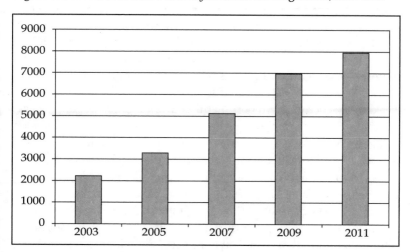

subjects including general knowledge, basic mathematics, Bangla and English.

Once selected, *shasthya kormis* undergo 12 days of training while staying at the BRAC training and resource center. The initial training focuses on health issues and technical skills. Sometimes program organizers also arrange for new *shasthya kormis* accompany an experienced *shasthya kormi* for a few weeks to observe and learn. While active, *shasthya kormis* join *shebikas* for the monthly refresher trainings. In 2009, BRAC began to train some *shasthya kormis* as skilled birth attendants. Over 1,200 have been trained and have begun to provide delivery services in the field (Zahan, 2010).

In general, *shasthya kormis* report that they enjoy the training and would in fact like to have opportunities for more, but for some, leaving home for the

Selection criteria for a *shasthya kormi*
• Female
• Secondary school certificate (10 years) (in particularly remote areas this is sometimes waived)
• Married
• No children under two years of age
• Lives in or near the catchment area
• Stable family life
• Age 20-35 years
• Willingness to receive two weeks residential and two weeks field training in the local work area
• Commitment for community work
• Community acceptability
• Motivated to help people

duration of training is difficult. Women who cannot leave their children at home often need to bring a child to the training center, in some cases with the accompaniment of a caretaker (often a mother-in-law). While BRAC allows *shasthya kormis* to come with children and caretakers, they charge them for room and board. This represented a significant expense for *shasthya kormis*.

Shasthya kormis are expected to work from 9AM-1PM six days a week. In practice, many report that they work more hours on average, particularly when including the time it takes to travel between villages. Unlike *shebikas*, who as volunteers have some flexibility if they decide to stop working, as paid workers, *shasthya kormis* are expected to be more consistent in their schedule. Each *shasthya kormi* supervises 10-12 *shebikas*, visiting them individually about once a month for two days at a time (see Table 6.3 for complete list of *shasthya kormi* activities). During these visits, she reviews their daily activity log and accompanies them to see any patients experiencing side effects or conditions beyond the *shebika*'s medical purview. The *shebika* will mobilize villagers to attend the prenatal care center and health education forum that the *shasthya kormi* conducts during her visit as well. Three days a week, *shasthya kormis* visit approximately 35 households each day, to achieve approximately 600 visits per month. On the other three days, they hold health education events, crosscheck *shebika* activities at various households, and handle referrals. The *shasthya kormi* serves as the first line of referral when TB patients experience minor side effects of treatment.

The *shasthya kormi* is not involved in financial transactions and communication between BRAC and the *shebika*; these are all handled by the program organizer. At times, the *shasthya kormi*'s authority over the *shebika* is a bit ambiguous. This arrangement can result in a lack of accountability or responsiveness, or it can allow for a very open communication that fosters effective partnership. Some *shebikas* see the *shasthya kormi* as a legitimizing presence for their work. One comments, "If she doesn't go to my area, people would not believe my work. If she goes, people might like her work and trust what I do (Zahan, 2010)."

Shasthya kormis also take on additional activities based on demand in the community. Selling medicines and attending deliveries are examples of two common expansions of their traditional activities.

Some begin to mediate marital issues, address issues of intimate partner violence, and advocate against sexual harassment within their communities (Zahan, 2010).

Table 6.3: *Shasthya kormis* scope of work

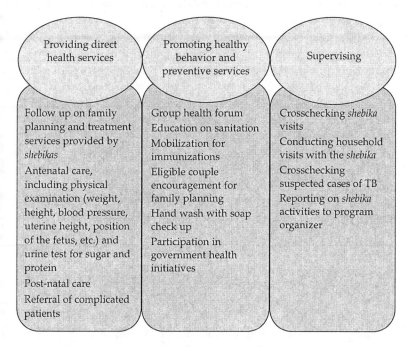

Providing direct health services	Promoting healthy behavior and preventive services	Supervising
Follow up on family planning and treatment services provided by *shebikas* Antenatal care, including physical examination (weight, height, blood pressure, uterine height, position of the fetus, etc.) and urine test for sugar and protein Post-natal care Referral of complicated patients	Group health forum Education on sanitation Mobilization for immunizations Eligible couple encouragement for family planning Hand wash with soap check up Participation in government health initiatives	Crosschecking *shebika* visits Conducting household visits with the *shebika* Crosschecking suspected cases of TB Reporting on *shebika* activities to program organizer

*Shasthya kormi*s report that antenatal activities take the bulk of their time, and running the health education forums tends to be their favorite activity. Administrative duties relating to *shebika* supervision are considered the most tedious tasks.

In contrast to the *shebikas*, there are no performance incentives for *shasthya kormi*. Each receives Tk 1200 (US $17.14) a month, which is considered an honorarium rather than a salary. They also receive a small stipend to support their travel for supervision and trainings. For antenatal care, *shasthya kormis* collect Tk 15 (US $0.21) for the first visit (village organization members pay Tk 10) and Tk 10 (members pay Tk 5) for subsequent visits. These fees are turned over to program organizers and absorbed by the essential health care program.

Interviews with *shasthya kormis* find that some supplement their income by selling medications or by making referrals to private facilities. Though they are instructed to only make referrals to the public facilities, the combination of reluctance from some patients and the promise of financial incentives for referrals from private facilities result in deviation from BRAC's policies by some *shasthya kormis* (Zahan, 2010).

Program organizers provide the primary supervision to the *shasthya kormis*, with each overseeing about four of them. Each month, they review the *shasthya kormi's* action plan, crosscheck her activities by visiting a few households at random, collect the money and compare it to her deposit records of antenatal care activities. Occasionally the sub-district manager will also conduct household visits to crosscheck her work as well.

Shasthya kormis have quantitative targets for their work, which many perceive as unrealistic. In the particular set up of BRAC's programs, *shasthya kormis* are highly reliant on the *shebikas* to meet their targets—in most cases, the identification of children in need of vaccination, pregnant women, and other populations of interest rests on the *shebika's* efforts; *shasthya kormis* with active *shebikas* will be more productive and likely to reach their targets. *Shebikas* are often aware of the *shasthya kormi's* reliance on their efforts. One reflected, "[the] SS's [*shasthya shebika's*] job is to keep the information of all the area, and SK's [*shasthya kormi's*] job is to maintain the link with us (Zahan, 2010)."

Shasthya kormis sometimes respond to the targets in adverse ways. Qualitative research conducted in 2010 indicated that they may inflate their monthly achievements. Some sold medication on the side to raise funds to hand over to the essential health care program to give the appearance of having done more antenatal visits than in actuality were conducted. In 2011, BRAC drastically reduced some of its targets to decrease the pressures on the *shasthya kormi* and create more realistic performance expectations.

Some managers report that high-performing *shasthya kormi*s have the necessary skills to become program officers. Most program officers are male, which as BRAC expands increasingly into antenatal care, creates some difficulties in supervising activities. *Shasthya kormi*s would largely be disqualified under the current requirements for program officers' educational achievement, so the program would need to adjust the criteria if they want to begin to draw from this pool.

Though not routinely evaluated, turnover among *shasthya kormi*s is a challenge, particularly in urban areas where women can find alternative employment opportunities that offer higher salaries. Qualitative studies indicate that the most common reason for leaving the position is remuneration, with other reasons including family illness, decisions to pursue higher education, and dissatisfaction with the position (Zahan, 2010). As mentioned in the discussion on *shebika* retention, turnover is costly in financial and quality terms, so BRAC must weigh these costs in determining a fair and effective compensation level for the *shasthya kormi*s.

6.11 Performance-based payment: When and how

"All systems are perfectly designed to achieve exactly the results they get."
—*Donald Berwick*

Pay-for-performance schemes in health care have attracted great praise and subsequent criticism in policy and academic debates. In this context, they generally are aimed at improving efficiency or productivity as there is an assumption that providers want to provide high quality care. Many studies note that when metrics are not perfectly aligned, they can create distortions and lead to unintended harm rather than improvement. Careful systems are thoughtful about the potential dangers that are being introduced and monitor them vigilantly. Though in informal conversations, BRAC's supervision system is often stripped down to simply its design of incentives, in truth, the *shebika* model contains intensive supervision, ongoing training and peer support, and linkages to a larger system (Figure 6.3).

The final level is through the use of process specification—that is, the implementation of mechanisms to ensure that pre-specified protocols are followed. These mechanisms focus on intervention at the point of decision-making, rather than patient outcomes. Monthly refresher trainings provide an opportunity for community health workers to re-familiarize themselves with the existing protocols and clarify areas of confusion or disagreement. Onsite supervision and crosschecking households are ways in which BRAC helps monitor the consistency of health delivery.

Figure 6.3:   Formal and informal mechanisms of support and supervision for *shasthya shebikas*

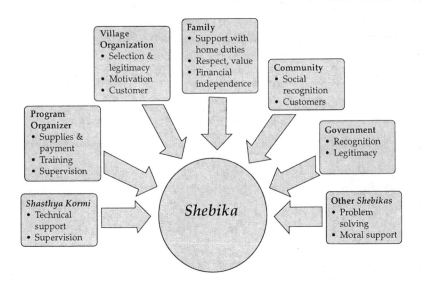

Why BRAC uses performance-based payment schemes

For most of its history, BRAC has been significantly self-funded. Its primary concern has always been scale, opting to provide a basic package of services for many versus an intense package for a few. Paying for results has allowed it to spread its resources more broadly than it would have done otherwise. As mentioned earlier, the cost of supporting a *shebika* after one year of training is roughly US $34 annually; it is only by achieving these levels of costs that BRAC is able to support a cadre of 89,000 *shebikas*.

BRAC wants the *shebika* to serve the needs of the community. They provide the training, the supplies, and the revolving fund to help her get started, but over time, her value to the village should sustain her livelihood. BRAC wants the *shebika* to see herself as accountable first to the community, not BRAC, and believes a salary would not support that dynamic. In addition, BRAC trusts that its frontline workers are incredibly innovative in experimenting with new strategies that increase their effectiveness (see Chapter 2 for a discussion of BRAC's use of financial incentives in its earlier programs, like OTEP). Paying for performance empowers and rewards volunteers to experiment continuously, relying on their own experience and knowledge rather than that of central office staff.

In BRAC's research and informal meetings, it's clear that *shebikas* want to become salaried workers. Most believe that they would better perform their work if they had a consistent income. While the comparative performance is debatable, there are many *shebikas* who struggle to provide for their families with the income that the position currently yields. Many of the best performing *shebikas* have significant support from a husband or a mother-in-law. These *shebikas* are effective, but they are not the poor and marginalized women that BRAC initially wanted to engage in the program. Conversely, one *shebika* in urban Dhaka, who could not afford her own mobile phone, spoke about begging to get the funds to call her program organizer or check in on patients. Clearly, these *shebikas* have motivation that transcends the simple monetary rewards that BRAC offers. The salary may enable them to be more effective and may reduce turnover for those who are on the margins. Salary and performance incentives are not mutually exclusive; BRAC may be able to find ways to compensate *shebikas* while still rewarding productivity.

The sheer magnitude of the shebika workforce means that the financial implications of committing to even a low level of recurrent compensation represent a significant responsibility for BRAC to consider. However, incremental changes demonstrate that this issue is being taken quite seriously. In 2011, *shasthya kormis* were granted additional benefits, including maternity leave and two bonuses annually.

Supervision and accountability

As discussed in Chapter 2, BRAC's initial experiments with community-based volunteers faced challenges with *shebikas* working to maximize their profits by selling as many products as possible. Its first strategy was to reduce the workforce only to those who seemed to be intrinsically motivated to keep patients' well-being in mind: namely, women. In addition, by placing the selection of the *shebika* in the hands of the village organization, BRAC creates a sense of local supervision and accountability—the *shebika* knows that the village organization expects her to serve the community appropriately and that they can call for her replacement if she takes advantage of her position.

BRAC's reporting system closely monitors and audits the activity of every *shebika* (Maher et al., 2003). In practice, however, the greatest accountability factor is the village. "Because villagers pay for her services, control rests ultimately with the buyer, rather than the purveyor (Smillie, 1997, 24)." The primary mechanisms are economic in nature, but significantly embedded in a social structure. When one *shebika* in Gazipur was asked what kept her from selling medications to more people, even when they didn't need them, she said, "If I get sick and need treatment, these are the people that I will depend on to take me to the hospital. If I've been cheating them, they will not help me!"

BRAC is careful in its processes. Only in cases when a patient is very ill can a diagnosis for TB be made without the patient giving at least one sputum sample in person at a smearing center. It's difficult to manufacture fake cases. *Shebikas* are expected to keep a log of all their activities, including which services were rendered at which household. *Shasthya kormi* often provide follow-up services to these same individuals. The proximity of the supervision and their familiarity with the village are also significant safeguards against misinformation.

Finally, for TB, BRAC has chosen an effective metric: patient outcome, confirmed by a sputum negative smear at the completion of treatment. In this case, the *shebika*'s best interest is perfectly aligned with that of the patient. By requiring it in person, identity is confirmed.

Another reason why this works is that generally, it's in the *shebika*'s best interest to treat as many patients as possible, thus encouraging active case finding and agreement to provide all patients with adherence support. Because it's unlikely that *shebikas* ever have more than a handful of TB patients under treatment, she has no incentive to avoid treating someone. Within a village, a *shebika* has a monopoly on BRAC's incentives, so she is best served by serving everyone.

6.12 Conclusions

Elements of BRAC's programs have relevance to community health volunteer programs elsewhere. With the health workforce shortage estimated at 4.3 million, there is an urgent need to experiment with and scale cadres of community health providers (WHO, 2006, 12). BRAC's experience indicates that in TB control, community-based activities can be particularly effective in identifying patients and ensuring high cure rates. While community-based health workers may have limited expertise, they are able to provide basic education, mobilize patients to seek diagnostics, provide social support and supervision for medication, and identify side effects that require referrals. Their ability to fulfill these functions effectively depends on their technical competence, motivation, and institutional support. BRAC takes care to adequately train, manage, and support community health workers to enable them to be effective agents of TB control.

In the past ten years, BRAC has tested whether its model can be adapted to contexts beyond Bangladesh (these are discussed in Chapter 8). Certainly the concepts of close supervision from field staff, regular training and group meetings, and monitoring of performance have relevance in all community-based field programs. In TB control, BRAC has implemented financial incentives for identifying patients and successful completion of treatment, and initial evaluations are promising.

It's important not to lose sight of the bigger picture when evaluating the *shebika* model. While immediate gains in health are one priority, so is broader societal change in gender equality. This type of impact takes time; what one observes in BRAC's current programs in Bangladesh is the result of over 30 years of experimentation and sustained efforts. The initial *shebikas* were not readily accepted, and the model challenged established power dynamics along professional socioeconomic, and gender lines. Community acceptance can take time, and discouraging results during the initial phases are not necessarily indicative of longer-term feasibility and effectiveness.

Reflecting on the program in a paper published in 2008, the authors note that, "BRAC's decision to switch to an exclusively female cadre of CHVs [community health volunteers] also exemplifies many of the complexities and contradictions about the often gendered nature of CHV programs. In a conservative social context, the choice reflects a strong cultural need for female health workers to provide basic services to women, while BRAC's transformative agenda has simultaneously focused on developing the skills and public roles of poor women through a longer process of community development via the VOs (village organizations). Empowerment in this public sense is linked both to this long-term process and to the significant scaling up of programs. The aim is to create new norms around gendered competence and public visibility (Standing and Chowdhury, 2008)."

These goals cannot be measured discreetly or in the short-term. Changing norms requires persistence and the willingness to sustain a model without the immediate results in hand. Certainly *shebikas* today enjoy much less resistance from their communities to their activities, and gender norms in Bangladesh are undergoing a larger process of transformation. For programs that want to advance values of social justice in their health programs, BRAC's experience can be instructive in helping programs have realistic expectations for the time required for these objectives and help them anticipate some of the early challenges that they may confront, such as BRAC having to grapple with the violence and resistance its first *shebikas* confronted from their villages.

Gains in other sectors open new doors for health delivery strategies. The idea of creating a cadre of *shasthya kormis* was implausible in the 1970s. Women did not have sufficient access to education to find such a qualified pool of candidates. Once the public sector achieved major improvements of educational attainment in women, BRAC could consider updating its strategy to strengthen its delivery systems. As *shasthya kormis* expand their technical expertise, they again come up against the boundaries of what the community accepts as their scope of work. Accounting for the time it takes at the village level for social norms to adjust and latent demand to be catalyzed will be important in tempering early program expectations and creating realistic performance targets.

BRAC's model requires a *shebika* to respond to the needs of her community in order to survive financially. In addition to all the technical aspects that BRAC must provide in order for the model to work, at the strategic level, giving the *shebika* the right basket of goods and services is crucial. Over time, the village needs evolve, new sources of competition arise, and buying habits change. BRAC must maintain a finger on the pulse of these trends, either by encouraging *shebikas* to make suggestions, or through other means.

Particularly in environments where BRAC has less intimate knowledge of the communities, as in Africa, utilizing mechanisms to respond to community health volunteer demand and feedback can improve the program effectiveness immediately as well as enable it to evolve. BRAC stands to gain from attracting and retaining talented volunteers. In order to achieve this, it must find a level of compensation that's competitive and attractive to its workers. Creating a motivated workforce will enable it to adapt continuously and maintain relevance.

Selected Photographs of BRAC's TB Program

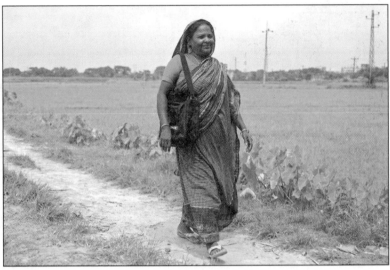

Photo 1: A BRAC-trained shasthya shebika *(community health volunteer) walks to her next client*

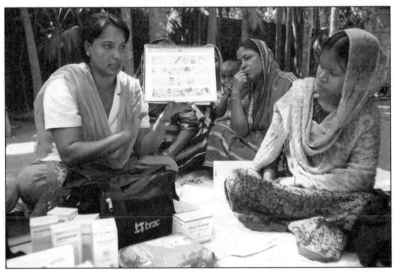

Photo 2: During a monthly health forum, the shasthya kormi *(health worker) teaches villagers about important health issues, like the symptoms of TB*

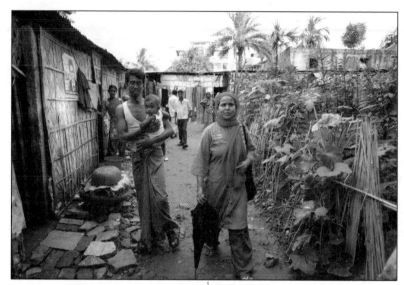

Photo 3: A shebika *goes through one of Dhaka's slums making household visits*

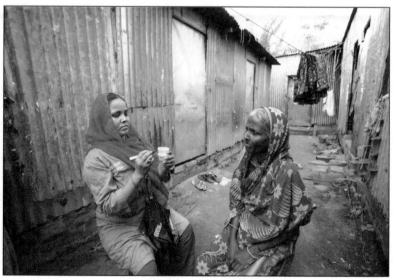

Photo 4: She gives a cough pot for sputum collection to a woman who has symptoms of TB

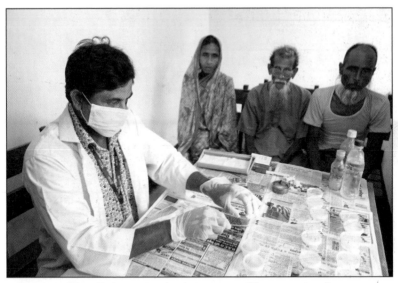

*Photo 5: A program organizer prepares slides at an outreach
sputum collection site*

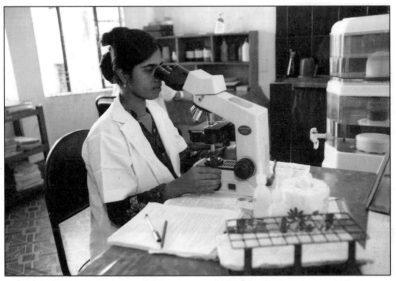

*Photo 6: At the BRAC laboratory, a technician performs microscopy to
look for TB bacilli*

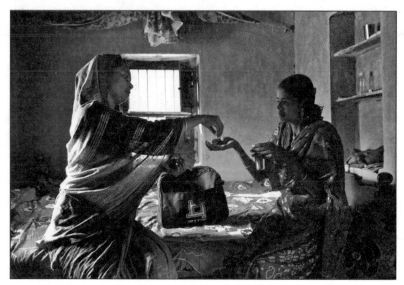

Photo 7: A patient comes to the shasthya shebika's *house every day to take medication under her watch*

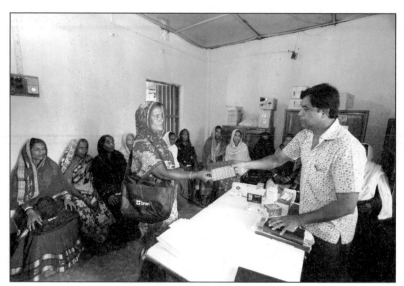

Photo 8: Shebikas *replenish their supply of medications and health products at monthly refresher trainings*

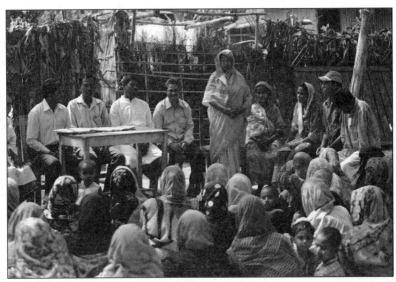

Photo 9: BRAC organizes community events with local leaders, shasthya shebikas *and cured patients to raise awareness of and reduce stigma around TB*

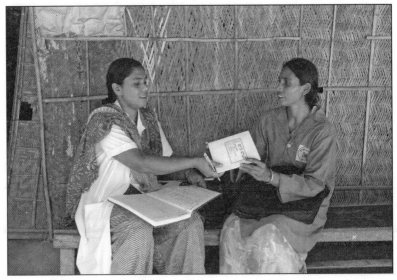

Photo 10: The program organizer reviews a shebika's *activities and supervises her performance.*

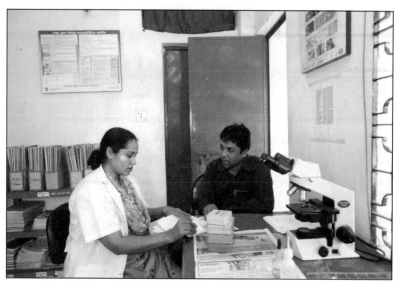

*Photo 11: Program organizers check the inventory of TB medications and
laboratory supplies in one of BRAC's branch offices*

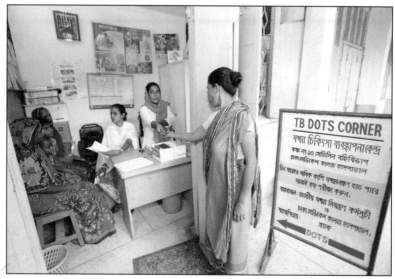

*Photo 12: BRAC's DOTS corner provides testing, referrals, and
treatment in hospitals and medical colleges*

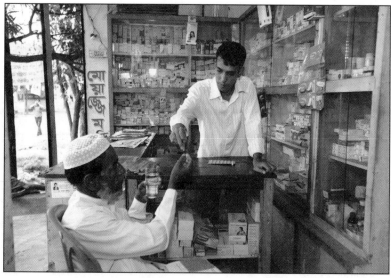

Photo 13: A BRAC-trained pharmacist provides DOTS to a patient living in an urban slum

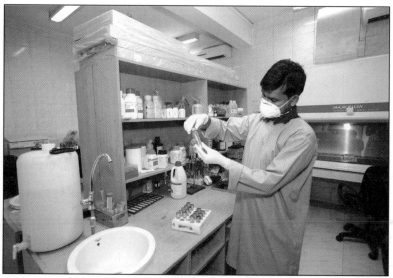

Photo 14: A laboratory technician at the National Institute of Diseases of the Chest and Hospital performs drug sensitivity testing

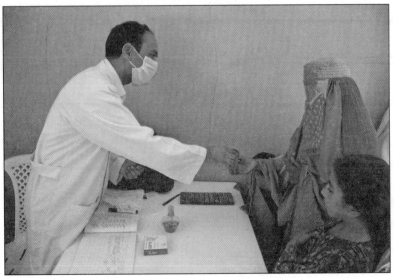

*Photo 15: An Afghan woman with symptoms of TB collects
a cough pot for sputum*

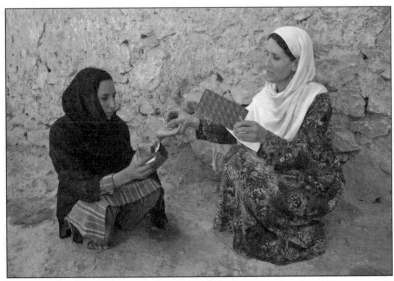

*Photo 16: A community health worker in Afghanistan provides
DOTS to a TB patient*

Chapter 7

Tuberculosis Control Strategies for Urban Bangladesh

"First I consulted the drug seller, and he gave me some medicine but I did not improve. After having symptoms for 15 days, I went to the chest hospital where the doctor gave me some medicine and ordered me to visit him at his private chambers. He called me there just so he could collect his fee; I gave him 300 taka and he prescribed me some more medicine. After I took it, my condition became worse. Then I visited another doctor, followed by yet another. Finally I was referred to BRAC [Dhaka Urban] by my neighbor."

–Male TB patient (Sherzad, 2008)

Questions of expansion are inherently complex. As discussed in previous chapters, there are many different modes of scaling up that organizations can pursue, each with a unique set of opportunities and requirements. In particular, once an organization has developed an effective program, the decision about entering a new context that would require it to start from scratch has significant implications. In the case of BRAC, "new contexts" existed domestically and abroad. The consistent trend of urban migration following independence changed the face of Bangladesh; by 2005, one in four Bangladeshis lived in an urban area. Dhaka in particularly had grown from a sleepy capital city in 1971 into a huge metropolitan area, with official population estimates around 9.1 million in 2005 (Angeles et al., 2009). It is one of the fastest growing cities worldwide, with a growth rate of 2.7% annually. Poverty is ubiquitous, and about 40% of the population lives in slums. Mobility is quite high and increasingly young women come unaccompanied from rural villages, motivated by the new levels of economic independence that the expanding garment industry provides. The social capital, local elite, and sense of village "eyes and ears" are largely absent; slums are often controlled by thugs and informal leaders, who frequently extort money from residents and shop owners, and for a significant population, moving is so common that they are termed "floating people." Establishing a TB program in a city like Dhaka poses a formidable challenge.

When facing these questions in the mid-1990s, BRAC also had to recognize that its identity had changed. It was no longer a fledging local organization, but one pursuing national scale in several areas. When planning for growth, it had new considerations such as its relationship with the public sector and the activities of the large number of other development NGOs that had moved into Bangladesh over the years.

7.1 BRAC's early urban programs

Establishing a footprint

In the 1990s, BRAC noted increasing mobility among individuals in rural areas and began to explore the possibility of setting up urban programs. In 1998, BRAC established microfinance programs in the slums of Dhaka (Afsana, 2010, 65). It also observed that the garment factories employed thousands of women who potentially could benefit from basic health services. It approached the Bangladesh Garment Manufacturers and Exporters Association (BGMEA), a group of factory owners that represented about 71,000 workers, to see if it could implement a basic health check-up model that it had briefly piloted in the Rajshahi city corporation, but never scaled up in other urban areas. BGMEA was supportive of the idea, and BRAC's program organizers began to visit the factories and provide basic screenings for eye health, reproductive health, and other issues. Program organizers were not trained to treat these conditions, but rather just ensure that referrals were made for those who required care. In this process, program organizers learned that many garment factory workers had not received their tetanus toxide vaccinations, and in many cases their children were not fully immunized. BRAC approached the city corporation with this information and learned that the city corporation was providing vaccination opportunities in the slums regularly, but that utilization was limited. BRAC began to recruit women from the microfinance groups to provide social mobilization for these services in 2000. Before long, BRAC decided to add the other components of the essential health care program and offer the basic check-up in all of BRAC's 32 branch offices in Dhaka.

Urban challenges with the shebika model

However, the urban context posed challenges to the *shebika* model that BRAC had not faced in rural areas. There was far less social capital in many neighborhoods; migrants tended to identify with their home villages rather than where they stayed and many moved frequently. They did not necessarily know the *shebika* and at times treated her with suspicion. While some reported that they did not confront challenges in gaining acceptance from their communities, others faced significant trials, including the need to correct misperceptions about her work. Afroza, a *shebika* in Badda, remembers, "It was very difficult for me when I first started. Many people in my community wanted to know why they had to pay for drugs, if BRAC got them for free from the government. And they didn't understand that I was a volunteer; they thought I was getting paid, so they didn't want to buy from me." Improving the community's perception required the *shebika* to make multiple household visits and efforts from the program officer to reinforce the information. In many instances, it was difficult to find opportunities for these interactions, as her neighbors often worked long hours and were not home during the hours when she typically conducted her household visits.

The pool of *shebikas* also had distinct characteristics from the rural areas. Many of the women in urban areas came for economic reasons, lured by the large number of new opportunities provided by the garment industry, and for the first time in Bangladesh's history, they came alone. Finding women who met the criteria for the *shebika* proved more difficult, and turnover rates were quite high. Particularly for the most competent women, BRAC's volunteer model could not compete with the wages available at the factories.

7.2 Early efforts to establish an urban TB program

Initially, the National Tuberculosis Program chose to focus its programming on the rural areas. Once coverage in these areas had been established, it began to tackle the challenge of urban TB control.

Bangladesh has six city corporations,[1] with Dhaka and Chittagong being the largest (see Table 7.1).

Since independence, migration to the cities had created continuous growth and pressure on limited public infrastructures. Massive slum settlements emerged, where migrants lived in relatively small and crowded quarters. Urban areas, and slums in particular, provided an ideal environment for the transmission of airborne diseases like TB, and the continual travel of migrants to and from their home villages threatened the gains that the rural programs had made.

Table 7.1: Population and slum characteristics of Bangladesh's city corporations, 2005

City corporation	Population, millions	% of population living in the slum	Overall population density (per km^2)	Population density in the slum (per km^2)
Dhaka metropolitan area	9.1	37	29,857	220,246
Chittagong	4.1	35	23,299	255,100
Khulna	0.520	20	20,346	132,988
Rajshahi	0.641	32	9,544	67,236
Barisal	0.351	30	7,152	133,730
Sylhet	0.756	27	12,961	154,741

Source: Angeles et al., 2009.

However, the goal of creating an urban response was complicated by the administrative system for health services in city corporations. Unlike the rural areas, in which delivery of health services was under the jurisdiction of the Ministry of Health and Family Welfare, city corporations had a chief health officer, who reported to the mayor on behalf of the Ministry of Local Government and Rural Development and Cooperatives. In the 1990s, as the urban population grew rapidly, it became clear that the demand for health services woefully overwhelmed the existing public infrastructure, and city corporations would be unable to respond on their own. The Asian Development Bank and United States Agency for International

[1] City corporations are urban areas that have their own governing structures and administrative services.

Development (USAID) independently began to fund two networks of NGOs to provide primary health care services in the city corporations.

The Smiling Sun Franchise Program included 27 NGOs that operated 323 static clinics and 8,500 satellite clinics in 64 districts, serving about 20 million clients (Smiling Sun, 2009). It was the largest USAID project in Bangladesh, providing a full essential delivery package along with safe delivery and diagnostic services (Urmee, 2011).

The Asian Development Bank-funded second urban primary health care project began in 1998 to improve the health status of the urban poor, particularly children. It provides essential and reproductive health services. Additional funding from the Swedish International Development Agency (SIDA), the Government of Bangladesh and United Kingdom's Department for International Development (DFID) also supports the project. Most of the services are provided for a fee, though the program strives for 30% of its patients to meet its criteria for free services (SUPHCP, 2011). Twelve NGOs deliver services in 24 reproductive health care centers and 161 primary health care centers, in total covering about 9.4 million people.

In 2000, the NTP approached the Dhaka City Corporation about establishing TB programs in the urban areas. "Urban areas lacked NGOs that had any previous experience in TB. In addition, primary health care activities in the city corporations were run by the local government. Determining how to best involve the city corporation health authority in the TB program was a major challenge for us," said Vikarunnessa Begum, who participated in these conversations along with Khurshid Alam Hyder, WHO, and Nobukatsu Ishikawa, Research Institute of Tuberculosis of Japan.

In the midst of these discussions, BRAC and the NTP were approached by a garment factory group, the Youngone Group, which was anxious to get a TB program for their workers in Chittagong underway. Vikarunnessa, Khurshid, and Ishikawa helped BRAC and the Youngone Group design its first workplace TB program and provided ongoing support during its first years. This experience helped the NTP see the value of working with NGOs and private sector partners in creating TB control strategies for Bangladesh's urban areas. They approached the Chittagong City Corporation and the primary health care NGO networks to discuss whether TB could be incorporated into their models. In 2001, urban TB control activities formally began in Chittagong.

In 2002, the Urban Primary Health Care Program and Smiling Sun Franchise Program began to establish TB programming in Dhaka, and in 2003, programming began in Khulna and other city corporations. Implementing NGOs entered a partnership with the NTP directly; the city corporations were not formally involved in the process.

7.3 Urban landscape for TB services

Figure 7.1: Options for seeking care for a cough in urban Bangladesh

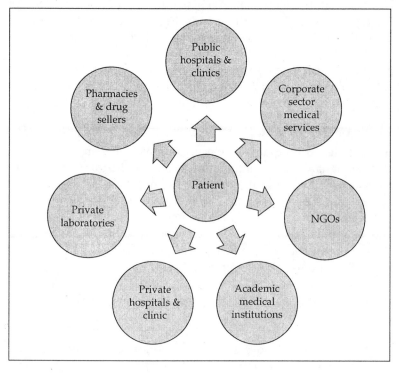

Note: Excludes restricted options, such as prison, defense and police medical services.

Source: Drawn from WHO guidelines for PPM (2008).

Policy makers had only sparse data and anecdotal observations to use in formulating a strategy for the urban areas. However, by simply mapping out the options, it was clear that the strategy would need to reflect the pluralistic landscape of other health providers (Figure 7.1). In terms of volume of care, the health sector was dominated by the private sector, with providers ranging from traditional doctors, drug stores and pharmacists, to sophisticated private hospitals. Private providers did not report their practices or treatment of TB, so the amount of TB being treated and patient outcomes were unknown.

Even within the public sector, hospitals lacked a designated program or clear treatment protocol. Patients were not offered DOTS or not followed through the course of their treatment. Many patients were not aware of TB or unable to diagnose their own symptoms as indicative of TB. Therefore, strategies to enhance patient ability to correctly identify their own condition would be a prerequisite to implementing stand-alone TB programs. In addition, since many patients were seeking care elsewhere, NTP needed to create mechanisms to move patients seeking care into the dedicated TB programs. Finally, improving care in the private sector would be necessary, as private practitioners would be likely to continue to serve patients that could pay without referring them.

Formulating a strategy

Similar to the division of rural areas by sub-district, NTP divides the city corporations among the NGOs by ward. It also designates specific NGOs to work with specific prisons, export processing zones, and factories (Figure 7.2).

In its 2005 proposal to the Global Fund (Round 5), the NTP proposed the establishment of a public-private mix coordination unit that would link its urban TB consultant with two coordinators (Bangladesh CCM, 2005, 134-135).This team helps NGOs strengthen their services and engage new partners, including private pharmacies, general practitioners, workplaces, and other stakeholders, including police, military, ports, railways, and academic institutions. The University of Leeds, United Kingdom also provided technical support and facilitated the process of engaging private practitioners in TB control in city corporations.

Figure 7.2: Conceptual diagram of institutions involved in national TB control activities

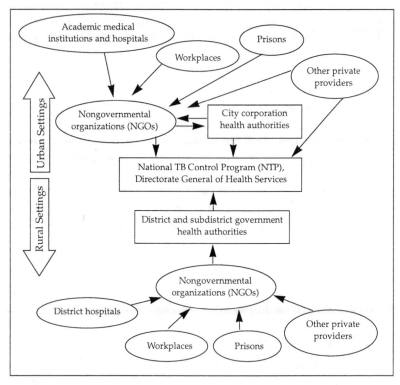

Source: Khan and Islam, 2010.

As with rural areas, the NTP allows NGOs to innovate on the service delivery to determine how to generate the best outcomes. NGOs are also given the bulk of direct service delivery and partnership-building activities. Ten new NGO partners that could strengthen efforts to reach new, non-traditional partners were recruited for Round 8. Five of these partners focus on intensifying community awareness and sensitization and do not provide direct services. Four others work in HIV and focus needs of patients living with TB and HIV and at-risk populations. The final partner is the Bangladesh Garments Manufacturers and Exporters Association (BGMEA), which provides TB services to factory workers.

7.4 BRAC's urban DOTS programs

In 2003, BRAC began to incorporate DOTS into its *shebika* programs in the peri-urban area surrounding Dhaka. These were densely populated areas where many migrant workers lived between the city corporation and district jurisdiction, and as a result had virtually no health system. Poised to establish these TB programs, BRAC decided that its programs in the city corporations were also mature enough to add this component as well. Laboratories were established in branch offices and *shebikas* were trained. It updated its memorandum of understanding with the NTP and the signed an additional memorandum of understanding with the city corporation authorities.

As in the rural areas, BRAC quickly became one of the largest implementers of TB services in urban areas. However, in the urban areas, BRAC realized that it would be unable to craft one delivery model that could handle the variable of the sub-populations and urban context. Instead, it created a portfolio of strategies to leverage existing health infrastructure, by improving quality of existing services and strengthening referral linkages. Its mix included establishing dedicated TB centers at existing hospitals, targeting garment workers, and reaching out to private practitioners.

DOTS Corners

In considering existing points of care, BRAC's leaders realized that the medical colleges were popular entry points, particularly for the poor seeking specialized care. These teaching hospitals were largely public but provided services at minimal costs. Quality was often a concern and a deterrent for some seeking care. However, they had the capacity to diagnose sputum-negative and extra pulmonary TB, both of which were critical capacities in scarce supply. They also saw a large volume of patients, providing the perfect opportunity for a diagnostic hub. In 2004, BRAC decided to create a dedicated "DOTS Corner" that would provide testing and treatment services, allowing patients to independently seek services and serve as a referral resource for physicians within the hospital. The new facility could also potentially leverage its own brand as a provider of DOTS services to counteract negative perceptions of the quality and efficiency of care delivered more generally at the hospital, persuading people with symptoms to seek treatment (Sherzad, 2008).

BRAC first requested that the NTP send a letter to the director of each medical college to introduce the TB program and urge the director to consider a partnership with NGOs to provide a dedicated TB program. As there was no overarching professional body, each college had the autonomy to respond independently, and in many cases, negotiating the initial agreement could be a lengthy process. When necessary, senior officials from the NTP met with the hospital leadership to explain the urgency of TB control to persuade them to partner with BRAC. BRAC also found that identifying an internal champion among the hospital's physicians was important in motivating referrals from all physicians, many of whom privately (or publicly) harbored doubts about the *shebikas'* ability to treat these patients.

Each DOTS Corner is maintained by a program officer and a laboratory technician. These women are salaried staff for BRAC; many worked in TB control in rural areas prior to the creation of the urban TB program and transferred in. They maintain the corner from 9AM-2PM, testing patients, providing DOTS to registered patients, and maintaining the registers. In the afternoon, they test the collected samples to identify new cases and often go out into the field to supervise local *shebikas*. A medical officer from the hospital confirms all cases prior to BRAC staff informing the patient. In 2011, BRAC has 12 DOTS Corners in Dhaka and 12 more in other cities (Table 7.2).

Table 7.2: **Patients referred and treated by BRAC DOTS' Corners, aggregated**

Year	Number of DOTS Corners in operation	Total cases diagnosed	Treated by the DOTS Corner (%)	Referred for treatment (%)
2007	22	8442	1100 (13)	7342 (87)
2008	22	9782	1180 (12)	8616 (88)
2009	23	11483	1344 (12)	10139 (88)
2010	24	11581	1283 (11)	10298 (89)

DOTS Corners also serve as hubs for all of forms of TB that require additional capabilities to diagnose, such as extra-pulmonary and sputum negative. While more difficult to diagnose, their treatment required similar daily support and supervision as new sputum smear positive cases. Over time, the DOTS Corners increasingly serve as a referral hub. After diagnosing a patient, BRAC staff discuss convenient treatment options with him or her and fill out the necessary referral paperwork so that he or she can begin treatment at the receiving center immediately. This model requires strong linkages between providers to ensure that patients are not lost between diagnosis and treatment initiation. Prior to 2003, these linkages were extremely weak and many patients were lost. Since the arrival of Global Fund resources and formalized relationships between the NGOs, these have improved.

Snapshot of a DOTS Corner: EPZ Hospital, Chittagong

The DOTS Corner opened in June 2005 on the first floor of the private EPZ hospital, which primarily serves the workers of the factories located in the zone. The DOTS Corner serves a population of over 100,000 that is served by 140 *shebikas* and 18 *shasthya kormis*, who, in addition to TB services, provide the full range of BRAC's essential health care package. It tests about 75 people a month and treated 175 patients in 2010.

Ishrat Hassain has worked in the DOTS Corner since its establishment and oversees the two other staff, as well as conducting field visits to supervise the *shebikas*. When she's in the DOTS Corner, she often receives calls from them regarding issues that come up in their work. She received training from the NTP prior to joining her post.

When they find a suspected case of TB, the shebikas will help the patients collect two sputum samples at their house, and then accompany them to the DOTS Corner for the final sample. The DOTS Corner also receives referrals from doctors working at the hospital. It is fortunate that one of the consultants formerly worked with BRAC's TB program and informally serves as a champion of the program, urging other physicians to verbally screen patients for TB regularly. About 10% of all suspected cases are referred by private practitioners, the largest source of referrals.

The DOTS Corner also holds motivational programs for factory workers, NGO workers, cured patients, and social leaders to raise awareness about TB and combat stigma. Ishrat notes that even now, stigma persists around TB, particularly for unmarried women, creating challenges for many to come forward for testing.

In May 2009, the DOTS Corner began to test its TB patients for HIV. Ishrat emphasizes the importance of counseling in getting patients to accept the testing, as they often are intimidated by the amount of blood that's drawn for the test. BRAC tested 112 patients in 2010. The DOTS Corner has also seen a few cases of multidrug resistant TB.

Creating targeted programs

Within city corporations, there are several populations that experienced a disproportionate risk of TB (Table 7.3). These include garment factory workers, prison populations, and slum dwellers, all of whom spent large amounts of time in poorly ventilated, crowded spaces. BRAC prioritized reaching these populations with TB services and has created tailored models to serve them effectively.

Table 7.3: Specific populations at risk in urban areas and BRAC's strategies to meet their specific needs

Who is the target population?	What are their needs?	BRAC's specific activities
Garment factory employees	Services that do not conflict with their work schedules; support from manager for treatment; privacy concerns	Sensitization of garment factory owners and managers Training for medical officers DOTS at convenient hours at nearby facilities, or via co-worker selected by patient

Provision of phone number on leaflets for confidential access |
| Prisoners | Onsite services; privacy/ stigma concerns services | Training for onsite medical staff; provision of drugs; testing |
| Slum populations | Limited mobility; transient lifestyle; poverty | Target typical first of contact— drug sellers, private providers Enable private providers to provide DOTS

Shebika-provided DOTS |

Garment factories

There are over 2.6 million workers in Bangladesh's garment industry, and 90% of them are female (Bangladesh CCM, 2007). In Dhaka, BRAC was given responsibility for 84 garment factories. At first, activities to build relationships with factory management were handled by BRAC's central office. Mahfuza Rifat managed BRAC's urban program and spent a good deal of time approaching factory leadership and onsite medical staff to discuss the

> "Much has changed since my diagnosis with TB. When I told my company I lost my job, because my boss said it was a contagious disease. Now I am unemployed and I am ill so I can't work."
>
> *Male TB Patient (Sherzad, 2008)*

risks of TB to garment factory workers and propose a partnership to provide TB control services.

Industry efforts to control TB

The Bangladesh Garment Manufacturers and Exporters Association (BGMEA) was established by garment factory owners to provide an organizing mechanism for the industry. As ready-made garments accounts for a significant portion of Bangladesh's exports, it is quite politically powerful.

Turnover of workers is a key challenge for factory owners. "These workers are the backbone of the industry. If they are not healthy, the wellbeing of the entire country is threatened," says Masud Quader Mona, BGMEA. BGMEA has opened 12 health clinics (10 in Dhaka, 2 in Chittagong) that provide free care for workers, and will soon have two hospitals as well.

In 2009, BGMEA and the NTP partnered to provide educational meetings to workers about TB. The following year, it signed a memorandum with BRAC to become a sub-recipient of Global Fund funding, and in September, the health clinics began to provide diagnostic services. To get services at the BGMEA facilities, workers are required to get a gate pass from their managers. The BGMEA TB control program has shifted from providing orientations for workers to focusing primarily on managers, recognizing the importance of buy-in at this level to effective TB control.

Once a patient is diagnosed, the health clinic begin to look for someone at the factory who can provide DOTS. Many factories have a nurse or medical officer onsite. In these cases, the TB control officer gives them a brief training on how to provide DOTS, and provides frequent supervision and support while they oversee a patient's treatment. If there is no onsite medical staff, the field officers finds someone in management to oversee treatment, or when necessary, a family member or other worker. Patients are required to have someone else engaged in their treatment at all times. As some factory health facilities are closed on weekends, some patients are given the weekend supply and expected to take medication on their own these days. Following patients for the full six months of treatment has proven to require significant effort from the program. Workers often switch jobs abruptly, so the TB program maintains frequent communication with them and their treatment supports, both in person and by phone.

Though efforts to diagnose and treat TB in factories have scaled, infection control efforts have not been implemented. The need is great. Each factory floor had approximately 200-300 workers. The BGMEA TB program lacks the resources to provide much active case screening. They encourage managers to be alert for workers with symptoms of TB and refer them for testing.

Urban BRAC programs serve many garment factory workers who prefer to keep their condition secret from their employer and co-workers. While those treated at BGMEA received two weeks paid leave when initiating treatment, those receiving DOTS elsewhere continued to work through this period.

BRAC provides training to factory medical staff on how to screen for TB. These patients are referred to BRAC labs for testing. In addition, BRAC educates workers about the risks and symptoms of TB. At informational sessions, it provides leaflets that could be distributed to other workers and include a phone number for follow-up questions. Many workers are quite concerned about confidentiality; because workers often live as well as worked together, the consequences for being diagnosed with an infectious condition can be severe. Factories can dismiss workers with TB as well, so many choose not to disclose their status to anyone. Workers often go to *shebikas'* houses early in the morning to receive treatment; they can also have it administered by the onsite medical staff, but willingness to pursue this option depends on the factory's attitude towards TB control. At Youngone Group, for example, all patients are required to take their medications in the morning from the medical center (Yesudian, 2007). The attending medical staff have received training from the NTP, and BRAC provides external quality assurance supervision for the laboratory.

Factories vary in their willingness to support TB control efforts. In some factories, including Youngone Group Limited, patients are given (mandatory) leave (usually without pay) for 2-3 weeks, after which they are no longer infectious and can return to work without endangering their coworkers. Youngone also explicitly states that employees cannot be fired because of a diagnosis of TB (Yesudian, 2007). Workers at other factories often do not have such protections.

In 2011, BRAC's central office staff is no longer involved in basic activities at the factories. Local branch offices have dedicated program organizers who visit factories every day. BRAC plans to engage another 150 new factories over the course of the year. Currently, BRAC's has directly engaged 185 factories in TB control.

Urban Slums

Forty percent of Dhaka's population live in slums (Angeles et al., 2009). Three large slums account for half the entire slum population, but there were smaller pockets scattered across the city. Residents of most small slums have created access to modern sanitation (a latrine linked to a sewer system or water sealed), but in the larger slums, it is rare.

Within the slums, pharmacies and village doctors, non-physicians who have completed six months of training, are common sources of medical services. In particular, people who are illiterate and women disproportionately seek out drug sellers as their first point of care (Sherzad, 2008). In many slums, BRAC had existing *shebika* programs, but found that these were insufficient to identify many of the patients with symptoms for TB. Therefore, it was important to engage the private providers directly. The Damien Foundation engages over 10,000 village doctors in rural areas in DOTS treatment with a cure rate of 90%, and the NTP had included its model in the national guidelines. BRAC aimed to draw on these same principles, though recognizing that in the urban areas, the density and fragmentation of the private sector required more intense training and relationship management.

> "Most people come to the BRAC center because there is no charge for treatment, and people prefer free services. We have also heard that the BRAC medicine comes from abroad, so the quality may be better than the drugs available in the market. Also, here the people take care of us properly and regularly—I could not take such care of myself because sometimes I would forget and fail to take my medicine. The BRAC center helps a lot."
>
> *Male patient (Sherzad 2008)*

BRAC provides quarterly trainings for pharmacists to attend. At the trainings, pharmacists learn about TB, the NTP-NGO partnership, national guidelines, DOTS, and existing programs where they can refer patients. Providers also receive posters to hang in their shops about TB and the phone number of a local BRAC program organizer in case they need new posters or any additional resources. Occasionally a village doctor serves as a DOTS provider as well, when a *shebika* was not convenient or a patient expresses a strong preference. Overall, *shebikas* continue to provide an important source of referrals and treatment support within the slums, particularly for the ultra-poor and vulnerable. In 2010, *shebikas* referred over 700 suspected cases of TB for testing. Government hospitals accounted for another 850, and referrals made to BRAC's Centers and private practitioners provided nearly 500.

Effective TB control also requires community-level activities to improve awareness and demand for TB services. BRAC recognizes that women often are unable to seek services without approval from their family, so creating acceptance and support for care seeking behavior is essential. BRAC holds quarterly orientations for opinion leaders and cured patients. When inviting opinion leaders to events, they stress that the TB program is led by the NTP, and BRAC is simply a local partner. A transportation stipend is provided. In 2010, 800 opinion leaders and almost 800 cured patients participated in BRAC's orientation sessions in Dhaka (Table 7.4).

Table 7.4: BRAC's social mobilization in Dhaka, 2010

Activities	No	Participants
Cured TB Patient	36	787
Pharmacist	12	261
Opinion Leader	36	800
HIV/AIDS NGO worker	13	282
Community Leader	2	44
Internee Doctors	2	252
Factory workers	84	4200
World TB Day	18	638
Review Workshop	2	133
Women 's association members	6	142
Cable TV message	12	NA

Prisons

Due to their crowded living conditions, prisoners are often at an increased risk for TB. They also lack access to the health system and require special onsite programs. With support from the NTP, in 2005 BRAC gained permission from the prison authorities to establish programs for inmates. By 2011, BRAC was working in the prisons of36 out of the 64 districts.

Each prison is supported by a DOTS Corner. A program organizer visits the prison twice a month to identify patients with symptoms and encourage them to provide two sputum samples. The prison's onsite medical staff, usually a medical officer or a pharmacist, is also trained in the symptoms of TB and can refer patients for testing. The program organizer transports these samples back to the DOTS Corner for diagnosis. When a case is identified, the program organizer informs the prison medical staff so that they can initiate DOTS treatment with medications provided by BRAC. During monthly visits the program organizer also follows up with the patient about their condition. Sputum samples at the end of the intensive and continuation phases are collected at the prison and tests at the DOTS Corner in accordance with NTP guidelines. If a patient is transferred or released during his course of treatment, the program organizer refers him to a local provider with the appropriate paperwork. In 2010, BRAC treated 224 cases of TB in prisons.

7.5 Challenges in 2011

BRAC's operations and delivery model

In all of its urban programming, BRAC treated 3,800 patients in 2010, with a cure rate around 90%. BRAC believes that there are a substantial number of cases that they were not identifying and continues to discuss potential strategies to create more access to TB control services.

> "When I first got TB, my husband started to hate me. When I came here [to BRAC] they told my husband that this disease isn't so dangerous, and it's curable. After becoming oriented with the program, his behavior with me has become normal again."
>
> *Female patient (Sherzad 2008)*

Urban areas pose a distinct challenge to BRAC because the clear need for segmentation of patients significantly diminishes the potential for scale. BRAC's urban programs are more intensive than its rural programs at both the field level and their need for middle and upper level management. Not only does the program require attention, but relationship management plays a large role in the ability of BRAC to effectively interact with other players in the larger health and social ecosystem.

In the field, BRAC suffers significant attrition in its *shebika* and *shasthya kormi* cadres. Program organizers in Dhaka comment that unless a recruit was "truly local," it was unlikely that she will last for too long. In some areas, they prioritize local commitment over other requirements and are willing to compromise on educational attainment, for example, for someone that they felt more confident to retain. While at times BRAC accepts unmarried candidates, as in the rural areas, these women often marry and leave shortly after beginning their duties.

In 2009, RED undertook a study into occupational exposure of TB infection among BRAC's health staff and volunteers. The results, which became available in 2011, demonstrated an elevated risk for TB infection, particularly among *shebika* with lower body mass indexes (Karim, Ahmed, Islam, unpublished). Many field staff express concerns about endangering their own health in their work activities, particularly as an increasingly number of MDR TB are diagnosed and treated without any additional precautions against exposure. "We are scared, but we cannot think about it too much, because if we aren't here to serve the people, who will be?" one *shebika* in Badda, Dhaka, asks. Many *shebikas* instruct patients to bring their own source of water when they come to take pills, fearing that transmission will occur if they share glasses with them.

Most patients in Dhaka with TB experience a significant delay (median 30 days) before diagnosis and initiation of treatment, creating a window for transmission to others (Sherzad, 2008). Delays are longer for smokers and those with a desire to maintain secrecy about his or her TB status. Compared to older studies, treatment delay has declined, but these findings suggest that there is need for more demand creation and strengthening of active case finding practices. While *shebikas* certainly can provide active case finding, as their workload increases, they may dedicate less time to this specific activity unless incentives or supervisory directives are instituted.

Ashar Alo Society

The Ashar Alo Society began as a self-help group in 1998. In 2010, it provided ART to 315 patients through three centers in Dhaka, Chittagong, and Sylhet, accompanied by support for prevention of mother-to-child transmission, treatment of opportunistic infections, and several types of counseling. Ashar Alo also provided prevention and testing services in the community.

In 2005, Ashar Alo joined the TB control partnership and in 2010 began to receive Global Fund funding from BRAC to provide TB services to its patients. All patients were verbally screened for TB during their appointments. When other NGOs identified cases of HIV, they referred the patients to Ashar Alo for all of their care.

In 2010, Ashar Alo treated 21 patients with HIV and TB, 16 of whom were cured and five who died.

There were promising indications that BRAC has garnered a positive image in its communities. Many referred patients come based on word of mouth rather than formal campaigns. When surveyed in 2009, patients listed free medication (79%) and reputation/perceived quality (74%) as their motivations for choosing BRAC as their treatment option.

City-level coordination

In Dhaka City Corporation, there are 139 TB service facilities. Sixty-nine offer diagnosis and treatment, and the remaining 70 are exclusively treatment centers. Twenty NGOs, including 14 that participate in the urban primary care projects, are implementing TB control programs. The city has 14 DOTS Corners, 12 of which are managed by BRAC.

Coordination is handled at the city corporation level. NGOs and the NTP hold semi-annual planning meetings; representatives from the city corporations or private sector do not typically attend.

At least once a year, all stakeholders involved in Dhaka's TB control efforts are invited to an urban DOTS meeting. In February 2011, BRAC and the NTP convened a meeting of all stakeholders involved in urban DOTS to correspond with Ishikawa and his colleagues' visit from Japan's Research Institute of Tuberculosis and Khurshid's visit from the WHO Southeast Asia Regional Office in India. Both the Research Institute of Tuberculosis and WHO provide ongoing technical support and a consistent presence in the partnership activities. NGO partners provided presentations of their programs and the NTP provided an update and summary of overall achievements. Private providers and the city corporation officials were not in attendance.

Participants used this opportunity to identify cross-cutting challenges and discuss how to address them. Some of the key challenges that emerged included: referrals, engagement of private practitioners, and increasing the case detection rate.

Table 7.5: Cases treated by the National Tuberculosis Program and its partners, 2005-2010

Year	All cases – national	All cases – urban	% urban
2005	122,298	22,485	18.4
2006	144,838	26,065	18
2007	147,448	26,612	18
2008	151,062	26,756	17.7
2009	160,735	28,156	17.5
2010	157,703	21,014	13.3

Coordinating HIV and TB treatment

Though HIV prevalence in 2011 was below 0.01%, many experts think there is potential for transmission to surge if preventive measures are not adequately instituted (WHO website, 2011). People living with HIV are at high risk for TB because of their compromised immune system.

With funding from the United States Agency for International Development (USAID), many TB programs began to provide HIV counseling and testing services in their facilities; by 2011, BRAC has established six centers, Damien Foundation has three, and the National Institute of Diseases of the Chest and Hospital has established one. BRAC tested 1,662 patients in 2010.

Transfers

A key component of the urban DOTS strategy is to create hubs for diagnosis that channel patients to convenient treatment centers. Patients receive a transfer form to take with them to the DOTS satellite center with the information about their diagnosis. Once they reach the other facility, the facility staff register them for treatment and send one portion of the form back to the referring institution.

Table 7.6: Feedback on referrals from the Dhaka DOTS Corner, 2010

Partner to whom a patient was referred to from BRAC DOTS Corner	Number of patients referred	% of referral slips that the DOTS Corner received
Government hospital	3069	17
BRAC DOTS Corner	1070	80
Other NGOs	1894	34
Total	6033	34

Patients can easily be lost between diagnosis and treatment. Currently, no direct communication between the point of diagnosis and care takes place; all information is transferred via the patient. Neither side systematically checks up on the patient to see if he or she follows up on the referral. If the patient loses the form, he could easily go elsewhere and get diagnosed again. Often the DOTS treatment centers are overwhelmed and the forms are not returned to the diagnosing site (Table 7.6). For the transfer system to ensure that patients do not get lost between diagnosis and treatment, the partnership needs to rethink this crucial linkage and how to strengthen it.

7.6 Conclusions

In many ways, BRAC's urban TB control strategy represents a major departure from its usual strategy of creating a model that can be widely replicated with little customization. BRAC's early experiences with health programs in Dhaka revealed the limitations that the *shebika* model would have in an urban setting. As opposed to rural areas that where there may be more limited numbers of health care providers, urban areas offer a wide range of options, with varying prices and convenience, to match the diversity of the city dwellers' needs and ability to pay. BRAC looked for existing leverage points that were underutilized in TB control efforts, such as public hospitals and medical colleges. As BRAC found in 2003, "DOTS Corners" offer an effective point for diagnosis, but their value multiplies when connected to a wide network for treatment facilities that provide convenience for patients. Similarly, private providers represent an important first point of care for many patients. Instead of competing with them, BRAC aimed to engage them in partnership. This is not an easy process, and BRAC still struggles with finding a systematic process to partner with private sector actors of all sizes.

Certain segments of the urban population are at increased risk of TB. The *shebika* model has limitations, particularly in reaching those who spend all day in a workplace outside of the home. BRAC has designed strategies to reach garment factory workers and slum dwellers that offer them convenient services for their lifestyle. Though significant inroads have been made in reducing stigma and TB-related discrimination in the factory workplace, for many garment workers, confidentiality remains a paramount concern. BRAC's ability to instill trust in patients is important in giving them the courage to pursue treatment. It also points to the value of building informal channels of referrals, such as those that it tries to create through the cured patients clubs.

While TB control in an environment like Dhaka requires these strategies, BRAC's urban TB control program is far more vertical than its rural program, both in terms of its isolation from BRAC's other health activities and the greater development platform. As TB control efforts evolve, BRAC will need to continuously balance the benefits of a targeted approach with the opportunities to respond to broader patient needs.

Effective partnerships for urban TB control

Leaders of the partnership acknowledge that they've yet to truly create TB control model that effectively covers all populations in

Bangladesh's urban areas. Efforts to engage partners need intensification and the mechanism tying together the program's many activities need strengthening.

The city corporation officials are notably absent from most discussions of TB control program planning and implementation, and the vast majority of the programming is implemented by NGOs, even within the public facilities. "It works for the time being, but nothing structural has been created," one WHO representative lamented.

What partners have clearly learned is that the complexity of the urban context requires them to create the right mix of several strategies, rather than focus on the development of a perfect model. Within the city, there are several populations with distinct preferences and care seeking behaviors that coexist. It is unlikely that all can be channeled to one source of care; instead, the TB control program will need to create TB programs that meet them at their current points of care, homes, or workplaces. Partners are thinking broadly about potential champions and partners, expanding their activities to engage industry partners, private practitioners, and other public sector units. However, the "private sector," often characterized as a uniform group of providers, has significant variations as well, from the independent drug seller with minimal qualifications marketing to slum dwellers, to the sleek franchises that appeal to the middle class. Even at the point of engaging private practitioners, NGOs and the NTP will need to think about how these different segments can be reached and enticed into the partnership mix.

Engaging private sectors, while crucial, will not create access for those who work during the hours at these facilities are open. Many urban dwellers work long hours and have difficult accessing services, putting their health and the health of their co-workers at risk. Initial activities to engage industry partners have been promising, and more is needed. As programs at BGMEA scale, they will need more support to manage the patient load, and NGO partners like BRAC will need to respond. In addition, participation is currently voluntary; policy-level change can serve as an effective mechanism to quickly catalyze changes in enabling workers to access TB and other important health services.

Many engage in ongoing experimentation and are working hard to develop models that allow for significant customization around an individual patient's lifestyle, needs, and preferences. To saturate the urban area, all of these activities are critically needed. The additional challenge for the NTP, BRAC, and others is to harness the variation and channel it into a well-coordinated system that can support patients in quickly accessing the support that they require. Unlike the rural areas, where NGOs can focus simply on their relationship with local public sector partners, the urban areas will require a much more cohesive frontline, indicating a need for more coordination mechanisms.

Chapter 8

International Experiences with Community-based Tuberculosis Control

8.1 Deciding to go abroad: Afghanistan

Recognizing that many of the problems facing Afghanistan in 2002 were not dissimilar to those Bangladesh confronted at its independence in 1972, BRAC decided for the first time to establish a presence abroad. Sir Fazle Hasan Abed, BRAC's founder and chairperson, recalls thinking, "maybe BRAC has some skills in getting people resettled and helping them get in developmental mode." Donors and policy makers approached Abed to request BRAC's participation in efforts to rebuild the nation. BRAC's initial assessment visits suggested that there was potential for BRAC's engagement. Relying on its own program funds, BRAC sent a five-person team to Afghanistan to implement the core package of its development portfolio: microfinance, education, and health.

Jalaluddin Ahmed, a member of BRAC's original assessment team, remembers, "We knew that setting up programs in Afghanistan would come with its own set of challenges. But we didn't know what they would be exactly." The team had no difficulty identifying areas of need and extensive challenges. Afghanistan had the lowest literacy rate in Asia; a mere 15% of women could read (Smillie, 2009, 227). Annual per capita income was US $230, under the international standard of extreme poverty (US $1 per day). Average life expectancy was 47 for men and 50 for women (WHO, 2008). No formal health system existed; health indicators were some of the worst in the world. Under five mortality was 200 per 1,000; diarrheal disease and pneumonia accounted for half of all deaths (WHO, 2008). Family planning had been banned under the Taliban and the fertility rate was close to 7 (Ahmad, 2004). The maternal mortality ratio was 1,400 per 100,000 live births. Furthermore, general infrastructure was in a similar state of disrepair. The transportation system was dismal. Good roads were rare, and in many areas, donkeys and horses were the only options available (Ahmad, 2004).

The team noted that Afghanistan differed from Bangladesh in many ways that they would need to consider. Afghanistan's population of 30 million was predominantly rural, like Bangladesh, but these rural dwellers were scattered much more sparsely, concerned about the threats of cold and drought, isolated by impassable mountains and extensive ethnic and lingual diversity (WHO, 2008).

8.2 Getting started

Few organizations were providing microfinance, and there was doubt that Afghan women had the requisite autonomy to participate. BRAC forged on nonetheless, incorporating the essential health care package into the model as well in three districts of Balkh province to evaluate its feasibility. Community health workers provided education on health and nutrition and sold ten basic health products for a small mark-up.

BRAC initially focused on creating the political and organizational relationships that would be required to operate effectively at scale, once the resources could be secured. Over the years, BRAC had provided informal support to other development groups in Afghanistan, and it approached these groups to learn more about the landscape. Within the government, BRAC was largely an unknown name. The team met with many public officials at the national and local levels to educate them about BRAC's experience and discuss how they could support the government's plans.

8.3 Afghanistan's basic package of health services

In March 2002, the Ministry of Public Health began to develop a plan to rebuild the country's health system. It identified the country's most urgent health needs, and prioritized creating broad access, including to residents in rural and remote locations. By 2003, it launched a health strategy called the basic package of health services

(BPHS) that would promote equitable access to health delivery by establishing a national infrastructure. It contained seven main components: maternal and newborn health; child health and immunization; public nutrition; communicable disease treatment and control (including TB); mental health; disability services; and regular supply of essential drugs (Ministry of Public Health, 2005). Basic health centers, comprehensive health centers, and district hospitals would be established. In addition to these facilities, the BPHS called for the creation of a community-based cadre of unpaid health workers that would serve in pairs (one of each gender) as a "health post," serving 1,000-1,500 population. The plan included specific details down to the number of staff, types of diagnostics, and list of medications that should be provided at each level. Recognizing that human resources for health were quite scarce, it set a target of one doctor or nurse per 10,000 people. Equity of quality and access between urban and rural populations were explicit goals.

The estimated cost for the program for the first seven years was US $1.4 billion to implement the program nationally (Ahmad, 2004). Donors, who were already facing the commitments they'd made immediately after the fall of the Taliban, were slow to meet this demand. Finally, in 2003, the United States' Agency for International Development (USAID) awarded the Ministry of Health US $35 million to initiate implementation of BPHS in rural and underserved areas of 14 provinces (Ministry of Public Health, 2005). Recognizing that there were many strong health NGOs working in Afghanistan, the Ministry of Public Health selected several to operationalize the plans established in their framework. As it anticipated, this strategy enabled a much more rapid scale up than the public sector could have achieved by working independently. By 2005, three quarters of the country had partners implementing the BPHS.

The introduction of BPHS marked a significant shift in how health NGOs operated in Afghanistan. It created expectations for their activities and incorporated them into a larger system, with a coherence strategy and set of national priorities. Implementation of BPHS would standardize health services and types of facilities nationwide, facilitating health system strengthening over time.

BRAC's activities under BPHS

In 2003, the Ministry of Public Health selected BRAC to begin implementation of BPHS in one district of Kabul Province. The following year, BRAC was successful in its bid to cover the provinces of Balkh, Baghdis, and Nimroz, with a population of approximately 1.5 million. One of its first activities was to establish health facilities. Often beginning service delivery in rented spaces, BRAC worked to build and renovate buildings to become the service delivery fully functioning facilities. In addition, it manages all aspects of health delivery, from hiring and paying staff to building the local supply chain. BRAC also provides significant training and technical support for other implementing NGOs.

Figure 8.1: BRAC's health budget in Afghanistan, 2003-2010

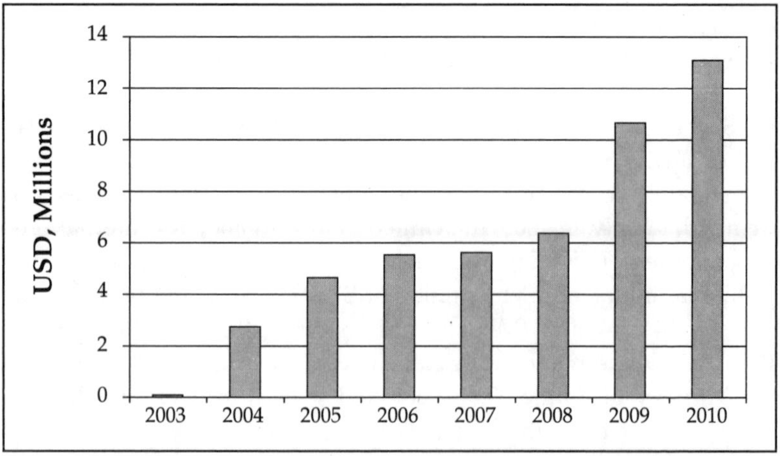

BRAC's health program scaled rapidly as a result the sudden availability of funds (Figure 8.1). From 2003-2004, its health budget increased from US $109,000 to US $2.7 million. BRAC's first priority was to create basic infrastructure at the community level. At the same time, it was establishing microfinance programs, enabling it to leverage the same platform that had proven effective in Bangladesh.

The CHW model as part of BPHS

A principle tenet of the BPHS was the free provision of basic medications and services to the Afghan people. The package created the position of a health post, which consisted of two health volunteers—one male and one female—for every 1,000-1,500 people. By 2011, BRAC had trained 5,700 community health workers to provide community-level access to basic services.

Community health workers are explicitly prohibited from selling medications. BRAC created a different set of incentive structures, using program funds, to emulate the pay-for-performance principles of the *shebika* model (patients receive the services free of charge). Some of its current incentives include:

- 60-100 AF (US $1.20-2) for attending monthly review session;
- 20 AF (US $0.40) per delivery;
- 2 AF (US $0.04) for condom distribution and 5 AF (US $0.10) for administration of injectable contraceptives.

While in many ways, the *shebika* model translates easily to the Afghan context, the mountainous terrain and limited population density create challenges for achieving full coverage. Whereas in Bangladesh, one *shebika* can cover 200-250 households, here a worker's catchment area has been reduced. BRAC was forced to scale its coverage expectations down to about 30-60 households. While the community health workers themselves did not receive a salary, the supervising program organizers did. An increase of this magnitude would be difficult for BRAC to support financially. The Afghanistan team decided to experiment with a hybrid technical and managerial cadre. They would hire women for a small salary (750 AF or US $15 a month) with higher levels of schooling, provide them with more advanced training, and have them act as a first tier-referral for the workers as well as a field supervisor. One community health supervisor oversees 10 workers, and one program organizer can then cover three community health supervisors and their 30 workers.

Under the BHPS, community health workers receive substantially more training than the *shebikas*. During their first six months, they receive 48 days of classroom training in 3-week blocks interspersed with two months of field activity. Following completion of these three intensive phases, they attend a review meeting each month. Community health workers cost the program an average of US $247 for the first year and US $83 in subsequent years (Reichenbach and Shimul, in press).

BRAC's criteria for workers in Afghanistan are very similar to those used in Bangladesh. Lower levels of education among women mean that the program has to be flexible on the requirement around schooling and account for very limited literacy in its training, data collection, and supervision practices. In general, Afghan health workers have less schooling and larger families than the *shebikas*. On an average day, most work for about three hours and visit five households. Much of their working time is consumed by travel. Most workers have no other form of income.

Unlike Bangladesh, where most *shebikas* compete with many other providers of health services, in rural Afghanistan, there are virtually no local options for health, public or private. Just 2% of workers indicate that there were other health providers in their area that diminished their sales (Reichenbach and Shimul, in press).

Despite support from the government for BRAC's efforts to increase community-based health delivery, there is continual debate around performance-based payments. The major question is: are incentives sustainable? For now, BRAC argues that they are essential for maintain an effective community workforce. "If you don't compensate them somehow for their efforts, how long do you expect them to keep volunteering?" Fazlul Hoque, BRAC, asks.

8.4 Community-based TB control

Like Bangladesh, Afghanistan is considered one of the 22 high burden countries for TB (Table 8.1). In contrast to the typical epidemiological patterns, more Afghan women are reported to have TB than their male counterparts.

Table 8.1: TB in Afghanistan, 2009 estimates

Incidence of TB (per 100,000)	190
Incidence (SS+ per 100,000)	79
Prevalence (per 100,000)	270
Mortality (per 100,00 population)	34
New MDR cases (%)	3.2
% of all cases in women	68

Sources: NTP, 2010 except for % of cases in all women, which is from NTP Afghanistan, 2009.

TB control was included in the BPHS, but DOTS was not a common practice. When patients were diagnosed, they were given a week's worth of medication at no cost, and expected to return weekly throughout the course of treatment. There was no active case finding or adherence support. BRAC thought that a *shebika*-like model could greatly increase case detection, particularly in women, and raise the cure rate. When BRAC approached the government in 2005 about piloting community-based DOTS, it found that the government officials were largely unfamiliar with the strategy. BRAC shared with them their experiences in Bangladesh, and a few senior Ministry of Public Health officials visited the program to see the model.

With approval from the government to provide DOTS at the community level, BRAC began to look for funding. FIDELIS, the Canadian International Development Agency's (CIDA) funding to the International Union against TB and Lung Disease for small pilots to boost case finding in underserved populations, had been an important supporter of TB programming in Bangladesh, giving BRAC's program several opportunities to experiment with its model. Akramul Islam and Rifat Mahfuza, who had overseen the BRAC's FIDELIS projects in Bangladesh, visited the Afghanistan program to help them design a project proposal that was appropriate for Afghanistan. In 2005, BRAC applied for US $174,000 to implement a range of activities. It received 15 months of funding beginning in January 2006 to pilot the program. Some of the initial goals focused on creating the infrastructure necessary to support the service delivery activities, such as establishing 50 new microscopy centers and conducting sputum smearing outreach. Mobile sputum smearing sites were set up periodically in remote areas to eliminate the need to go to a health facility for diagnosis or during treatment, as sputum tests were recommended by the NTP at months 3, 5, and 8. From the mobile sites, BRAC staff could transport the slides to a microscopic laboratory for reading. The laboratory technician notifies program organizers about the test results, who shared the information with the community health workers so that they can initiate treatment.

BRAC also trains many health providers on TB and DOTS, including over 2,200 community health workers and close to 100 private practitioners. Many providers are unaware of the free services available for TB and how to help patients access them.

> "Following completion by the patient of the first phase of tuberculosis treatment at the health facility, the CHW should ensure compliance of TB patients with the second-phase treatment course in the community, based on DOTS. The CHW should create awareness among the community on how to prevent TB and should refer suspected cases to a health facility."
>
> *BPHS guidelines*
> *(Ministry of Public Health, 2005)*

At its one-year mark, the initial pilot yielded promising results. Case detection tripled in 2006, from 17% to 70%, and treatment success, already high at 85%, increased marginally to 87%. FIDELIS agreed to provide US $447,000 for an additional 18 months of activity, beginning in July 2008. The additional resources would allow BRAC to replicate many of these practices in other areas.

8.5 Scaling up DOTS nationally

In 2005, facility-based DOTS was added to the BPHS guidelines (Ministry of Public Health, 2005). In the same year, Afghanistan's Ministry of Public Health received funding from the Global Fund and several bilateral donors to strengthen TB services nationwide. By 2006, over 500 facilities had the capacity to diagnose TB and 900 provided TB treatment (ACCM, 2007). The Afghanistan National TB Program (NTP) estimated that it had established a DOTS center in almost every health facility (97%) (ACCM 2009). The program treated over 25,000 patients with a 90% cure rate, but it was clear that services were largely inaccessible to the rural and remote populations.

Prior to applying to FIDELIS, BRAC had received endorsement from the NTP on its proposals. During the pilot implementations, it shared the results with the public sector officials to alert them of the promising findings. In 2007, the NTP included community-based DOTS as an intended strategy in its proposal to the Global Fund and in 2008, added community-based DOTS to the initial phase of treatment in the national guidelines. The proposal also included plans to expand the sputum smearing outreach centers to remote areas in other provinces.

In 2008, Afghanistan applied to the Global Fund seeking additional support for its TB and malaria programs. Through a competitive bidding process, the Country Coordination Mechanism (CCM) selected BRAC to serve with the Afghanistan Ministry of Public Health as principal recipients for the TB proposal. Prior to submitting the proposal, the Ministry of Public Health decided to have BRAC serve as the sole principal recipient for TB control. In addition, BRAC was successful in its bid to be one of three NGO principal recipients in the malaria proposal.

In April 2009, Afghanistan received US $39 million for TB control activities from the Global Fund (GFATM, 2011). BRAC sub-contracts to the National TB Control Program and five NGOs. With these funds, community health workers receive the US $1 incentive for each referred suspected case of TB that is confirmed and US $3 for successfully overseeing a patient's DOTS treatment. BRAC is responsible for implementing DOTS in 11 of the 34 provinces (12.2 million population). The 19 other BPHS implementers are incorporating community-based DOTS into their activities in the remaining provinces.

Prior to Global Fund resources, BRAC's budget for TB-specific activities had been quite limited (Figure 8.2). In 2008, it had received less than US $130,000 for TB, forcing it to focus on implementing TB services within the BPHS funding, rather than focusing on developing more effective strategies. In 2009, with US $1.6 million allocated directly to TB, it was able to scale and strengthen community-based DOTS programming significantly. In addition to the workers, additional community mobilization activities were introduced.

Figure 8.2: Resources for health and TB in Afghanistan, 2003-2010

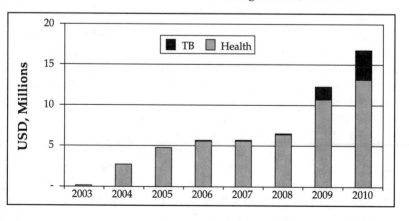

Strengthening community-based TB service delivery: the CAP Project

The TB Control Assistance Program (CAP) is a multi-country, USAID-funded project to strengthen National TB Programs. On the ground, it often is described as "filling the gaps" by providing technical support and resources for activities that are not covered by the Global Fund, particularly in the areas of capacity building and community-based programming. In Afghanistan, the primary objective of TB CAP has been strengthening community-base programming. TB CAP activities in Afghanistan began in 2008 and were managed by an American NGO, Management Sciences for Health. BRAC was one of the 14 BPHS-implementing NGOs selected as partners. It planned to pilot its activities in four districts in 2008, then scale up to an additional nine districts in 2009.

NGOs hold regular meetings to discuss progress and plans. In addition, within their respective provinces they are expected to engage with the provincial and regional TB coordinators. Coordination is particularly important, since in many cases, BRAC is implementing community-based DOTS through TB CAP in an area where another NGO provides BPHS. To avoid duplication, BRAC, provincial public health officials, and the other NGOs signed memorandums of understandings and communicate frequently. All stakeholders also attend regular review and coordination meetings at the central level.

Refining delivery strategies

To boost health worker morale and performance, BRAC decided to experiment with non-monetary rewards for facility-based staff. In three provinces, the team publicly recognizes its best performers at every level of service delivery, from the laboratory technician to the doctor to the nurses, and gives them gifts, including a blanket and pair of shoes, as a token of appreciation.

Through TB CAP, BRAC also expanded other types of activities at the community level to increase awareness about and demand for TB services. In 2010, BRAC conducted a 2-day DOTS training for 2,100 of its community health workers. These community health workers have held almost 5,000 meetings. In addition, BRAC expanded its community awareness activities to better reach key community figures. It organized over 100 educational meetings with Imams and 30 meetings at schools. BRAC also reaches out to traditional healers and village doctors to educate them about TB and the DOTS strategy.

Other efforts to increase case detection are initiated by the NTP. When a new case of TB is identified, the patient is asked to bring his or her close family members to the facility or community health worker for a verbal screening. In facilities that have implemented the health management information system, this is now a required entry, and supervisors follow up with facilities that do not report contact screening. BRAC screened over 17,000 contacts in 2010.

8.6 National TB control activities

Table 8.2: National TB control achievements, 2009

Total cases detected	26,358
Sputum-smear positive, new (new SS+)	12,497
Sputum-smear negative, new	6,108
Extra-pulmonary	5,730
Relapse	1,082
% of new smear-positive cases diagnosed in women	68
Notification rate (SS+ and overall, per 100,000)	53, 58
DOTS case detection rate (new SS+, %)	70%
DOTS treatment success rate (new SS+, %)	87

Source: Afghanistan NTP, 2010.

In 2009, 26,000 patients were treated for TB (Table 8.2). The national cure rate for new sputum-smear positive cases was 87%. BRAC's program treated 4,981 cases in 2010, and had a case detection rate of 70% and cure rate of 84%. Almost 70% of its patients are female.

Results from Afghanistan's first survey of knowledge, attitudes, and practices (KAP) on TB indicate that more education on TB and available services is greatly needed (Delawer et al., 2011). In general, Afghans consider TB a grave health concern. Most know that it could be cured, though they are unaware of how TB is diagnosed and the government's provision of free treatment. Levels of reported stigma and alienation are high; respondents themselves admitted that they try to avoid interacting with TB patients. Almost half believe TB is a female-specific disease (Delawer et al., 2011). Respondents were reluctant to seek care, preferring to treat symptoms at home, but if necessary would go to the government facility (75%). Many mentioned concerns about costs and geographical distance as deterrents to accessing care. Many of these findings point to the need for increased community-level service delivery and education.

Delivering TB control in the context of Afghanistan has required choreography between many stakeholders. Though the National TB Program has little involvement in financing or monitoring activities, it has provided clear guidance on how the program should be implemented, expectations, and the integration of TB control activities into larger health priorities. Afghanistan's political system is still gaining legitimacy in society, and there are many fragilities and tensions that make it difficult for the public sector to deliver services. NGOs are widely perceived as a more neutral party, and may provide an effective holdover measure while greater issues of governance are tackled.

The Ministry of Public Health and the NTP have showed an openness to innovative strategies to improve TB control. After BRAC demonstrated the efficacy of community-based DOTS and mobilization activities in its FIDELIS pilots, the NTP codified many of these practices in their national guidelines. A similar willingness to explore task-shifting in other critical areas, such as laboratory technicians, has led to a new cadre of high-school graduates that are trained in basic microscopy.

With regard to TB control, huge strides have been made in creating a national infrastructure. BRAC supports the NTP in managing the national supply chain, and facility-level stock outs have virtually been eliminated for TB medications (Global Fund, 2010). Remote areas still pose significant challenges for managing a robust supply chain; keeping facilities stocked with reagents and films can also be a challenge (Global Fund, 2010). BRAC is assisting the NTP in establishing four referral laboratories with the capacity to conduct drug sensitivity testing, including one in Herat that has already begun. Current estimates around multi-drug resistant TB indicate a rate of 3% in new cases, but the data are limited.

There are promising signs of system-level improvement. Not only are new capacities being created, but important quality mechanisms are also being institutionalized. For example, 80% of facilities submitted quarterly reports on time in 2010. The TB program met its 2010 target of having quarterly supervisory visits with documentation in at least 55% of facilities (407/714). In addition, external quality assurance measures have been established, and three quarters of facilities now undergo regular checks on their smear microscopy (Global Fund, 2010).

Some activities have proven to take more time than initially anticipated. Many of the challenges lie in reducing the barriers patients face in accessing treatment, with more activities needed at the community level and in private sector engagement. In 2010, just 20% of TB patients received community-based DOTS, and only 250 of the planned 1,000 private providers were partnering with the NTP (Global Fund, 2010). In addition to BRAC's 5,700 community health workers and approximately 2,000 volunteers providing DOTS in areas with another BPHS implementer, other NGOs now have 32,000 community health workers trained in DOTS.

Resources for TB control

Despite huge needs for TB control, absorptive capacity has created a challenge for taking advantage of international resources. Afghanistan first received funding for TB control from the Global Fund for 2005-2009 (Round 4). The approved amount was US $3.5 million, though only US $2.7 million was disbursed. In 2009 (Round 8), the Global Fund approved another proposal for US $10.2 million for TB programming 2009-2013. The program's expenditure rate is close to half of its projections.

In some cases, donors have noted the challenges and opted to modify their time horizons to account for the challenges in implementing intended programs. For example, TB CAP was initially scheduled to end in 2010, but due to under-spending, programming was extended until mid-2011. USAID opted to continue these activities in a subsequent project, called TB-CARE 1. BRAC will continue to play a large role in community-based DOTS activities.

8.7 BRAC Afghanistan in 2011

On the cusp of its 10-year anniversary, BRAC Afghanistan boasts a comprehensive portfolio of development programs and has become the largest NGO in the country, with a budget of US $36 million. Its microfinance program operates in 20 provinces, with over 200,000 clients. Given the low literacy rates and school enrollment rates for girls, education has been another priority of BRAC. Though many parents are reluctant to send their daughters to school, BRAC's 3-month curriculum and partnership with the World Food Program that enables them to provide meals creates a relatively attractive option. BRAC uses an intense curriculum to teach at an accelerated rate, so that the students are prepared to jump into the formal school system when it opens in the spring. BRAC has established 4,000 community-based schools that serve over 100,000 students. In additional, BRAC has established an "Adolescent Development Program" to provide vocational training for young women for whom higher educational options do not exist. The health budget accounts for a third of BRAC's in-country spending.

Human resources

Individuals with the qualifications to manage programs or deliver health services are scarce in rural Afghanistan. In addition, BRAC's relatively modest pay scale makes it difficult to compete with other international NGOs. As a result, BRAC sends staff from its Bangladeshi office to Afghanistan. Jalaluddin Ahmed, initial head of BRAC Afghanistan, spent five years onsite to develop the program. As in Bangladesh, most staff are based in the field. Speaking local languages is essential to creating a relationship with communities, and Bangladeshi staff working in Afghanistan are expected to learn basic Dari.

In BRAC's expansion in Bangladesh, building capacity at the local level enabled a great deal of decentralization of decision-making, crucial when rapid response and flexibility are required. Building a cadre of local leadership in Afghanistan is an important step in the program's maturation. BRAC has integrated this objective into many of its practices. For example, it supports its staff in seeking opportunities for graduate studies. Several promising staff went to Bangladesh to complete their graduate studies at the James P. Grant School of Public Health at BRAC University. BRAC established three training centers that offer courses to BRAC personnel and staff from other NGOS and the public sector in a range of topics.

When Bangladeshi staff run programs in Afghanistan, they are paired with a junior Afghan staff member to whom they provide on-the-ground training and supervision. Over time, the junior staff members gain the skills and experience to fulfill the position independently, and the need for the Bangladeshi manager subsides. Whereas in 2002, all senior positions were filled by Bangladeshis, currently all positions have been replaced by Afghans except for the country head, finance manager and monitoring manager.

Security and other challenges

Afghanistan is considered one of the most risky countries in the world for aid workers, so security concerns play a role even in mundane decision making (Walt, 2009). For example, when purchasing new vehicles for staff to move around the provinces, BRAC opted to buy used cars to reduce the chance of having them hijacked and stolen. These types of details can be easy to gloss over when decisions are made by headquarters staff who lack the daily reminders of the realities of the context. Establishing leadership for the BRAC program in-country minimizes these types of oversights, which can lead to inefficient utilization of resources and even potentially endanger local staff.

BRAC's greatest protection may come from its relationships with communities. Even when asked to move for security reasons, staff are often reluctant to leave a community where they have deep relationships and know that others will look out for them. In many areas, BRAC feels confident that it has won the support of the communities; they know that BRAC came for the long-run and are working to empower them. One staff member commented, "When I'm traveling, I feel insecure. I don't know the people on the way. But I know that once I reach the community, if anything happens, the people will save me."

8.8 Government partnership

In Afghanistan, TB control is a concerted effort by public and private partners, much like Bangladesh. However, while TB control in Afghanistan falls largely with the purview of the BPHS, it is embedded into a general set of health services to a much greater extent. This centralization of policy development enables an integrated approach. In the context of a country where NGOs deliver the vast majority of services, the standardization that the BPHS creates across geographies and partners facilitates equity in service delivery and efficiency in health system strengthening. Including TB control within this larger initiative creates a risk that it will not receive the necessary priority to successfully address the issue. Increasingly, the NTP has incorporated more dedicated activities to bolster the efforts, offering a compelling example of how vertical programs can complement a primary care approach.

BRAC is an international NGO in Afghanistan, so the dynamics of government partnership differ from its experiences in Bangladesh (Chowdhury, Alam, Ahmed, 2006). As a newcomer it had to prove its commitment and value, but can more easily maintain an image of political neutrality. Programmatically, BRAC has had much less latitude than it enjoyed in Bangladesh, as the Ministry of Public Health of Afghanistan has provided a clear directive and policy with the BPHS. However, BRAC has found that by demonstrating through pilots the power of community-based TB control activities, it has been able to convince the government to adopt some of its practices into the national guidelines. While implementation may have been slower or more restricted than BRAC's approach in Bangladesh, this experience offered unique benefits as well: these practices will now be implemented nationally by many other partners, achieving far more impact than BRAC could on its own.

8.9 Early efforts with TB control in Uganda

BRAC entered Uganda in 2005 and initially focused on building its microfinance, health, and agriculture programs. In health, it focused on creating a cadre of community health promoters (based on the *shebika* model), who delivered health messaging and health products within communities. Similar to Afghanistan, the Uganda program realized that household coverage would need to be pared down to be manageable for the workers. In rural areas, it was usually around 100, but in the more densely populated towns, one health worker could cover as many as 200 households.

The program decided to experiment with performance-based incentives for program assistants (similar to program organizers in Bangladesh). Their monthly salary is based on how many of their promoters were active, as defined by identifying pregnant women, treating illnesses in children under five, and selling health products. These metrics are independently verified by the monitoring team.

Though there was great reluctance from many senior and junior staff alike about implementing this system, the results have been compelling, and there are plans to enact similar systems in the agriculture program.

In October 2010, the World Health Organization's TB REACH project created an opportunity for BRAC to pilot DOTS treatment in the African context. BRAC began to recruit staff and establish laboratories in four districts of Uganda (population 1.7 million). Its primary strategies are the same: conduct semi-active case finding in the community, provide outreach sputum smearing centers to facilitate convenient diagnosis, and increase education and mobilization activities in the community. Incentives are provided to promoters for case identification and treatment. The program link with the public sector's health centers for referrals and laboratories when possible. These referrals are particularly important in Uganda because BRAC has not explored programming in HIV. Co-infection is an important issue that the promoters are not yet equipped to address. BRAC's integrated programs do not work in every village in Uganda, so in many places BRAC is training a woman in the village solely on TB services. The government has not allowed BRAC to implement the patient bond.

BRAC established a control population to compare its program to the existing system (facility-based DOTS with no community-based case finding). After six months, 433 cases had been identified in control areas, compared with 1,957 in BRAC's areas. BRAC ran a number of radio spots, street drama, and health education sessions to create more demand for TB services. Based on these results, the Uganda's National TB Program has recommended BRAC as a sub-recipient of Global Fund resources in the next proposal, which will enable it to expand. Members of BRAC's TB program in Bangladesh visit the program regularly and will support the scale up with their expertise.

8.10 Conclusions

This chapter offers a brief glimpse of BRAC's experience in TB control in Afghanistan and Uganda. BRAC's international strategy reflects its experiences in Bangladesh: take an integrated approach to scale (this will be discussed in Chapter 9). With minor exceptions, TB control remains embedded in a larger basket of activities for a community health volunteer, whose activities link with BRAC's other initiatives within the community. These core principles remain quite strong across BRAC's international portfolio and contextualize the smaller adjustments that have been made to the TB control model specifically.

For many countries, TB is a public health priority, and BRAC's community-based model has particular value in areas where health system infrastructure is still developing. DOTS is an effective strategy, particularly when daily support is convenient, which is rarely true for rural dwellers in the countries where BRAC operates.

When BRAC enters a new country, it assesses the context comprehensively to evaluate how it should adapt its programs locally. It considers the political environment, the health system, resource availability, other providers, and unmet needs. As it begins to plan its programs, BRAC looks for ways to take advantage of what exists, through partnerships or other strategies, and make its programs additive to others. These are examples of what local adaptation entails. BRAC's models cannot be imported in from Bangladesh and replicated without refinements. The guiding principles remain, but the activity system from country to country varies significantly. For example, BRAC has been unable to export the concept of the patient bond to Uganda or Afghanistan due to objections from the government, and its workers in Afghanistan are prohibited from selling medications. The impact of these modifications on patient adherence and health worker income (and consequent satisfaction and turnover) must be carefully evaluated. As BRAC pilots new strategies, such as a cadre of health workers in Afghanistan, new lessons learned that can be applied back to the original model can be identified: *Shasthya kormis* are an imported concept that has been fully integrated into community-health programming in Bangladesh. As BRAC's TB program scales in Uganda, it will need to account for co-infection with HIV, giving BRAC new insights into the applicability of the *shebika* model to other chronic diseases (Chapter 10 for exploratory remarks on this topic). More immediately, Uganda's early experiments with performance-based incentives for staff may prove effective in other countries as well.

Chapter 9

Growing BRAC: Management at Scale

> "I realize that trying to describe BRAC is like being one of the proverbial blind men trying to describe an elephant. Each description differs, depending on the part that can be touched. To make it more difficult, and at the risk of stretching the analogy too far, BRAC is like a moving elephant. Not only that, just when it seems the elephant has reached maturity, it grows again, so no description remains accurate for long."
>
> *Ian Smillie (Smillie, 1997)*

In Bangladesh, BRAC health covers over 110 million people with its basic essential health coverage program, provided by the *shebikas* (BRAC, 2011). Ninety-one million are covered by BRAC's TB control program. In addition to its current portfolio of TB, malaria, maternal, neonatal and child health, nutrition and sanitation, it's exploring new areas of health insurance, eye care and HIV-TB co-infection. Over 89,000 *shebikas* are active in the field, each supported by *shasthya kormi*s, program organizers, and higher-level project infrastructure and staff. BRAC Health's expenditure in 2010 was Tk 3.4 billion (US $45.4 million), just 12% of BRAC's overall expenditures. BRAC's education, microfinance, legal advocacy, and agricultural programs represent other significant levers for poverty reduction that have potential synergies with the health program.

Though large, BRAC as an institution is anything but static. Its leaders are ambitious and aggressively push the organization when they see a good opportunity. However, strong leadership is only one ingredient of maintaining excellence in results and practices over time. Many organizations falter as they scale up from failure to invest in the management and bureaucracies that big institutions require to function. Despite its community focus, BRAC has aimed for a sense of corporate professionalism in its work and borrows many of its practices from the private sector, where Abed worked prior to starting BRAC. Many have noted its uniqueness in this approach. For example, *The Economist* recently described it as "the largest, fastest-growing non-governmental organization in the world—and one of the most businesslike (*The Economist*, 2010)." To manage size and growth simultaneously in relentless pursuit of economic development, in the midst of changing landscapes, an organization requires strong leadership and a robust operational structure to support its activities. In addition to its programs, BRAC has developed a supportive infrastructure of mechanisms to house financial and human resource functions, as well as a separate monitoring branch to look after all the programs.

BRAC's brand is built on its ability to deliver quality results at scale with strong mechanisms for accountability. The systems are crucial, as they ensure that activities align and further BRAC's goals. But they only serve to provide operational effectiveness. It's strategic vision that creates a compass for BRAC's trajectory, and the translation of the vision into a coherent set of activities that determines BRAC's survival over time. Bangladesh is a quickly changing landscape and BRAC must keep pace if it's to remain effective. This challenge requires some programs to scale up, others to scale down, and still others to begin at the pilot level. And ideally, these processes would take place simultaneously and continuously.

> "Scaling up helps sustain the intellectual and physical growth of the organization. It raises the morale and motivation of the staff as there are more opportunities to be promoted; this also attracts 'brighter' people to join the organization, and aids in improving its overall quality. A large organization with successful programs draws the attention of the experts, policy makers, and the media from within and outside the country, which in turn increases the credibility of the organization in the eyes of these people and their constituencies."
>
> *Chowdhury and Cash, 1996, 42*

9.1 BRAC health program's value proposition

The ultimate customers of BRAC's health activities are the individuals that access its services. The *shebika* model offers a first stop for basic health needs of unbeatable convenience. It also creates linkages from the community to the health system to assist individuals seeking medical care in a more timely fashion. Some of these linkages are to BRAC's other programs, such as the prenatal care centers staffed by *shasthya kormis*, or to mobilization efforts, like the government's vaccination campaigns. Individuals also have opportunities to learn how to improve their health behaviors and access preventative products through the *shebika*. These health services are further integrated with other initiatives, such as microfinance and education, so consumers can access a broad range of services from one provider: BRAC.

Strategy and operational effectiveness

Classically, strategy involves the decisions around how to achieve an organization's goals. Michael Porter from Harvard Business School offers five tests of a good strategy for firms, which have some relevance for social organizations as well (Porter, 1996):

1. Unique value proposition (what is the benefit being provided that's distinct from what others are providing?)

2. Tailored value chain (how are activities designed and performed to maximize the benefits that are delivered?)

3. Activities that fit together and reinforce each other (how is the organization and infrastructure arranged to support activities?)

4. Trade-offs and choosing when to say no (how does the organization remained focused on its primary activities?)

5. Continuous improvement of realization of strategy (how does the organization improve its programs over time?)

Strategy drives the development of a program's road map, but for most organizations, resource constraints are significant. The goal of operational effectiveness is to achieve the optimal allocation of resources for a program. Issues such as right mix of staff skills, procurement policies, and quality assurance are examples of areas that, while not of direct strategic concern, certainly have an impact on an organization's performance. The danger of focusing just at the operational level is that there will be no vision, just a well-run machine, and as health needs and contexts evolve, the organization will cease to have its relevance to its communities.

While it's easiest to think of strategy and operational effectiveness as distinct, in practice overlaps are not uncommon. For example, as Faruque Ahmed, BRAC, describes the decision to create the cadre of *shasthya kormis* in Bangladesh, one sees aspects of both:

"We wanted to hire more program organizers but we didn't have the funds. With the increases in education, there are a lot more women in the villages that are available to work, but because there aren't jobs, they are housewives. If we give them an opportunity to work, not only do they help their community, but everything that they learn has an impact at home. Their family and the community benefit enormously."

While for the individual customer, the scale of BRAC's program may not matter, it is BRAC's ability to provide this service to such a large number of communities that makes it unique. In addition, household recognition of the BRAC brand creates a trust that legitimates the *shebika*, enabling customers to have confidence in her training and the quality of her products. The economies of scale achieved by the program size also lead to lower prices on health products and medications.

In order for BRAC's health program to maintain its value proposition, it must:

- Understand the community's most urgent health needs and assess the best tools for intervention
- Maintain a convenient "one-stop shop" at the community level with quality assurance and social legitimacy (e.g. the BRAC "brand")
- Reinforce linkages to the health system and other non-health programs

These tasks imply that BRAC must anticipate changes in, and maintain an intimate knowledge of, village life. It also must create synergies between programs and with other partners. Also, while preserving the BRAC brand and benefits of scale, it must decentralize decision-making to a level that allows *shebikas* to adapt the model to the specific needs of their communities.

Clearly, a well-articulated strategy and superior execution are required for BRAC to achieve these objectives. BRAC's leadership and management system are tailored to enable a dynamic mode of operation that can evolve with Bangladesh's needs. This umbrella enables specific programs, such as the TB control program, to thrive, while also ensuring that it is embedded in larger initiatives to capture potential leverage points.

9.2 Choosing activities that build organizational capabilities

BRAC has been described for decades as "a learning organization." Certainly its leaders like to consider it a dynamic organization. But what does it mean to be a learning organization, or dynamic? These characteristics develop over time from a mix of primary activities. Therefore, in designing its operations, BRAC needs to think about what capabilities it needs to be most effective and align its activities with these goals. Capabilities are often marginalized in explaining successful models or "best practices," as they are often more difficult to observe and develop over time.

But particularly for an organization with as many years of experience as BRAC, considering the capabilities that have emerged through decades of learning and growing is important in explaining its current performance. These capabilities may have important implications for other organizations that want to replicate BRAC's programs.

Figure 9.1: Activities create capabilities

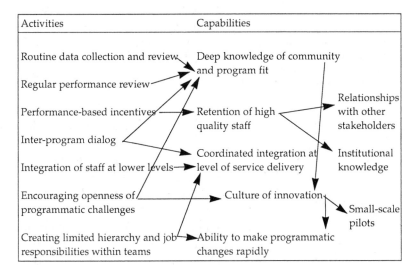

Through its practices, BRAC builds individuals and programs with extensive capabilities, enabling it to perform activities more efficiently or strategically.

9.3 Leadership within BRAC Health

"Our founder is a visionary thinker, born entrepreneur, and most importantly, an institution builder. BRAC is a dynamic organization, but one with discipline. When we're making a decision, we have lots of meetings, solicit a lot of feedback from the field, but once a decision is made, everyone gets moving on it."

Faruque Ahmed, BRAC

While long-term success requires more than strong leadership, BRAC certainly could not have achieved such tenure and program success without its truly exceptional leader, Sir Fazle H. Abed. Particularly in the context of a country undergoing constant change like Bangladesh, having a leader with the discipline to constantly assess the frontier and the insight to know which changes BRAC should respond to is a crucial explanatory factor for BRAC's trajectory.

At 75, Abed remains at the helm to provide BRAC with the same inspirational vision that brought it to life in 1972. He meets with the program directors regularly and consults with them about the strategic direction of their various programs. The consistency of his leadership has allowed BRAC to grow under a steady hand. In 1980, one researcher wrote, "Abed's leadership style encourages open discussion of difficult issues and acceptance of apparent issues, yet provides firm decisions when they are needed (Korten, 1980)."

> **Loyalty to a mission**
>
> "We have a very focused mission: the only kind of work we take up is connected with the lives of the poor. You are nearest to the mission when you're in the field, with poor people. Our staff working in the field are reminded of our mission every day. Our mission is very active; in fact it's built into the way we work. While project proposals are being written, we tend to find an answer to a particular problem through poor people's own agency. So when we talk about TB control we think in terms of a shasthya shebika as the answer to the problem. Even the way we design the program keeps us wedded to our mission."
>
> *Sir Fazle Hasan Abed, BRAC*

One of the greatest pressures facing Abed is his sense of how much remains to be done and all the areas in which BRAC is still needed. There is a constant internal push for BRAC to take on more—from creating a teaching hospital in Dhaka to expanding internationally.

Within the health program, BRAC has had significant stability in leadership, with Sadia Chowdhury serving from 1991-1998, and the current director, Faruque Ahmed, joining in 2002. The length of tenure has allowed for a longer arc in planning and strategy. In addition, many project managers have also made life-long careers out of their work at BRAC, some staying with a program from inception, others joining in one department and transitioning to others as new positions open up or are created. "One great thing about BRAC is that if you're willing to work hard and take initiative, there are lots of opportunities to get involved" says Mahfuza Rifat, who joined the TB program as a training specialist and now manages directly under Akramul.

Figure 9.2: Basic management structure of BRAC's essential health care program

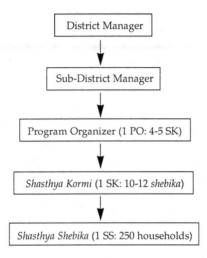

Program managers have significant autonomy in how they run their teams. As a result, effective managers need a blend of skills that included not only technical expertise, but also the ability to listen and communicate with staff.

BRAC strives to help talented staff advance within the ranks while also recognizing that fresh perspectives are also important for organizational health. Current managers represent a mix of individuals whose careers have grown with the organization as well as some who first had great achievements in other settings, such as the World Bank and in private sector information technology.

9.4 Integrated and vertical program organization

What the patient sees of BRAC health is the *shebika*, who provides an integrated range of services and products. Program integration continues up to the sub-district level, with staff allocating their time between the various demands of the different health programs.

BRAC has a local office in each sub-district where it works that houses all local staff for its programs (Figure 9.2). Program organizers provide supervision to the field staff. They and other staff manage the medication inventory, prepare the quarterly reports, and coordinate the monthly refresher trainings. At this level, most health programs do not have a dedicated staff person, except for those that require local technical expertise, such as TB.

At the district or regional level, where BRAC has another office, staff are largely responsible for supervising activities at the sub-district level. The area manager visits the various offices regularly to discuss any challenges. Some programs, such as the TB program, also have a dedicated staff person at this level that can provide technical support and monitoring.

At the central level, there is a core essential health care program, with other teams devoted to targeted programs, in part due to the nature of donor funding, which is usually project-based, and in part based on the specific program needs. Some projects, such as TB and malaria, are further sub-divided into clusters, such as those working with other partners and those focused on BRAC's implementation. Many of the staff at this level have completed a graduate degree in medicine or public health.

For the most part, there is little hierarchy within these teams. While each person has a specific scope of work, in practice team members must be flexible and comfortable performing a range of tasks, addressing needs from the field, preparing reports and proposals, attending to visitors, supporting government activities, or responding to donor requests requires efforts from the full team.

In 2010, BRAC had over 4,000 full-time staff in its health program, with just 70 based centrally (Table 9.1).

Table 9.1: Characteristics of BRAC health program's staff composition and structure, 2010

Number of branch offices	2,360
Number of field staff	3,972
Number of central office staff	70
Number of staff with graduate level degree (e.g. MD, MPH, etc.)	40

Resulting capabilities

While BRAC's staff roster is full of talented individuals, staff members comment that there is a mentality that "no one is indispensable." Creating a team approach to the work ensures that all members develop a range of general skills in addition to their existing technical expertise. Therefore as specific members leave to pursue education or seek opportunities at other organizations, rarely is there a loss of a specific skill set. The set-up also enables programs to rearrange dynamically as the specifics of program activities change and new central level activities are required. For example, when Akramul received a fellowship opportunity with the International Union Against TB and Lung Disease and spent two years based in New Delhi, the team was well prepared to manage the activities in his absence.

BRAC expects staff to continuously identify program weaknesses and make improvements. Even senior leaders maintain a critical lens. Abed says, "Making programs more effective is an ongoing quest for BRAC. We are always looking to find ways to continuously improve program quality and outcomes."

9.5 Centralization vs. decentralization

"Field staff will do the best job that they can. But we have to give them the right level of support and direction in order for them to be effective."

Akramul Islam, BRAC

A question facing all large programs is to what extent decision-making should be centralized versus delegated to regional or local managers. Centralized decision-making can lead to greater efficiency and standardization, but for projects where local specificity is required, giving field staff the autonomy to adapt will facilitate customization. These decisions stem from the top-level leadership, which has the most comprehensive perspective of BRAC's activities and strategic direction. However, it's important to note that managers at all levels face daily choices and trade-offs about how to allocate resources and time. Widespread communication of BRAC's strategy provides a framework to guide lower-level decision-making and over time supports alignment between frontline operations and central office planning. Korten writes, "BRAC's responsive style of programming has emerged within the framework of well-developed management systems designed to facilitate decentralized operation within a strong but evolving policy framework (Korten, 1980)."

BRAC centralizes many activities, such as supply chain management, monitoring and evaluation, and development of training curriculum. However, it encourages field staff to innovate locally. BRAC seeks funds for small-scale experimentation within its programs. In the TB program, the FIDELIS grants have provided resources for experimentation that allow BRAC to continue to refine the model while simultaneously implementing through the much larger and more rigid Global Fund grant.

Decision-making at the head office

Rapid decision-making is a crucial skill for a program of BRAC's size. Much of a program director's day is consumed with the miscellaneous but pressing issues that come in from the field. Program managers meet monthly to discuss any cross-cutting issues, but often hold more informal meetings weekly or even daily as a result of the high level of program integration and shared activities.

Directors from all programs also meet weekly to discuss inter-departmental collaboration. These are opportunities to discuss cross cutting issues and opportunities, such as risk management or investing in new technologies in the field. It also serves as a forum to discuss organization-wide changes or ways to facilitate collaboration between departments. As directors are often to represent BRAC at public events, these meetings give them a general sense of the major activities in other departments, better enabling them to speak comprehensively about BRAC.

In the 1990s, the health program invested in process documentation to capture process evolution real-time. As the program has grown, these documentation processes have subsided. However, in 2004, BRAC invested in an electronic management information system. All TB program data is now entered in the central database.

The management information system gives program managers the ability to integrate data into their action planning much more readily. For example, Akramul can look at sub-districts to determine which areas are in need of additional support from the central level.

Difficult choices

> "One of BRAC's biggest difficulties is to say 'no' when approached by a government department or a donor with a pressing need. BRAC cannot do everything."
>
> *Ian Smillie (Smillie, 1997, 47).*

While BRAC's achievements are great, the organizational culture tends to focus activity on the latest challenge and how much is left to be done. BRAC's leaders face this pressure from themselves, their staff, and outsiders on a daily basis. Choosing where to focus BRAC's efforts is essential to maintaining program quality, but the choices of when to say "yes" and "no" can be difficult. In fact, leaders within BRAC have noted that failing to say "no" is where BRAC gets itself into trouble. At times, emergent opportunities can drive BRAC's strategy, instead of a reflective strategy driving BRAC to find those opportunities. "The other issue that you need to talk about within BRAC is what do we really want to do? It seems that anyone comes with an idea and some money, and we start implementing without really looking at whether it is a priority, whether it will have an impact on the other programs, or the longer-term issues. That's the choice that we have to make," Mushtaque, Rockefeller Foundation (formerly BRAC), reflects.

When assessing a new idea for BRAC, Abed first thinks about whether the organization has the human resources to take it on. If so, he then begins to consider whether the financial resources are available and what future availability would look like, particularly for health projects.

As BRAC has emerged on the global scene and gained international recognition for its work, these pressures have only increased. Donors and organizations entering Bangladesh often seek partnerships or BRAC's leadership on new initiatives. With the emergence of new issues in global health, such as non-communicable diseases, universal health coverage, and mobile health, BRAC will need to consider how these resonate with its mission and own priorities.

There are several ideas that BRAC has investigated that it chose not to implement for various reasons. When approached by one partner about launching a line of franchise clinics for primary health care, BRAC felt uncertain that it had the appropriate staff to manage the initiative. Or, when the Bangladesh's Country Coordinating Mechanism (CCM) was first applying for HIV funding, BRAC opted not to compete for the role as a principle recipient, feeling that it would be overwhelmed by the responsibility that would entail.

Even at the individual level, leaders also face regular decisions about where to spend their time. Senior leaders are often asked to speak at international conferences or participate in various high-level committees. These opportunities are important ways in which BRAC can disseminate its lessons learned, increase its visibility to potential donors and partnerships, and influence global policy, but they also represent additional responsibilities that compete with the day-to-day management that the program requires. Creating a right balance is an ongoing challenge for all senior program leaders. Increasingly, BRAC as an organization is seeking to disseminate its work more broadly.

9.6 Human resource policies and retention

Accountability has always been a central operating principle for BRAC and is formalized in its management policies. All staff receive annual performance reviews with their supervisors and twice-annual bonuses based on their achievements. Informal feedback is provided regularly as well.

Turnover of staff is a recurrent area identified as a major challenge for service delivery organizations. At the program organizer level, BRAC sees significant turnover when the government issues a large recruiting order. Otherwise, its staff at the field, sub-district, and district level remains fairly stable. Despite the challenges in turnover, BRAC has high expectations for its staff and expects them to demonstrate their competency. All new program organizers go through a one-year probationary period before gaining full recognition and benefits. Central-level staff report that on the whole, program organizers are incredibly dedicated to their work. "They go above and beyond their job requirements to accomplish tasks. They really put a lot into making the program run." Rifat, BRAC, comments.

BRAC has created a culture of openness around programmatic issues. Staff are generally proactive about contacting supervisors about operational challenges. When it comes to giving feedback on management and relationships with superiors, however, there is far less openness. Managers sometimes solicit opinions from their colleagues, but there has been less investment in creating norms around this type of dialog.

At the central level, finding enough highly qualified people with management skills is always a challenge, particularly in times of growth. At times, programs will compete internally for the best staff members. In addition, BRAC must compete with international NGOs, many of whom offer higher levels of compensation. Increasingly,

BRAC is investing in its junior program managers to build a deeper bench of team members with management and leadership skills. In addition to technical expertise, communication and an ability to motivate one's colleagues are skills that BRAC emphasizes.

As Bangladesh's situation evolves, leading programs inquires increasing levels of technical skills. "The new health programs that are needed now often require significant technical expertise—it's not like oral rehydration therapy, where anyone can do it," Mushtaque comments. "Human resources are a real challenge." Increasingly, BRAC's ability to launch new programs is dependent on finding someone with the expertise to run them.

Doing by doing, or.....

"Sometimes we forget that we don't have to do everything ourselves. The TB program is a good example of how we can make sure that other NGOs are involved. There's a level of convenience in doing it ourselves; it allows us to control it. Partnerships have a higher risk; there's a greater chance of failure. But when you succeed, the magnitude of the success is much greater than it could have been if you'd done it alone" Mushtaque Chowdhury, Rockefeller Foundation (formerly BRAC).

BRAC uses a number of different strategies to scale up its programs. These include:

Program expansion: for many of its programs, BRAC has opted to scale up internally and manage the program itself. Often this is the fastest way to grow.

Government partnership: Increasingly, BRAC's programs are conducted in partnership with the public sector. In Afghanistan, BRAC manages the delivery of public sector services for several provinces.

Training others on the model: BRAC teaches other organizations about its model, usually by bringing them onsite to see it first-hand, and occasionally provides technical support.

Hybrid: As the situation evolves, BRAC's strategy can as well. Prior to the earthquake in Haiti in 2010, BRAC was providing technical support for a livelihood program. After the earthquake, BRAC felt compelled to contribute directly and built a limb and brace center.

Diffusion: BRAC also hopes that others will adopt its innovations more broadly, perhaps even without direct communication. In Bangladesh alone, there are 600 NGOs delivering non-formal education. Community health volunteer programs are implemented widely, and increasingly, there are programs replicating BRAC's strategy of targeting the ultra-poor in a number of countries. Consequently, BRAC seeks opportunities to share its delivery model so that others can incorporate appropriate elements into their own programming.

The recognition that the shortage of qualified staff was creating a bottleneck was part of BRAC's motivation to establish the James P. Grant School of Public Health at BRAC University. Since opening its doors in 2005, the school has produced approximately 25 graduates a year, primarily from the region. Many of these alumni are now employed by BRAC in Bangladesh and in its projects abroad.

9.7 Learning organization

David Korten, who spent time at BRAC for the Ford Foundation, suggests that development programs must engage in several distinct types of learning. In looking at successful cooperative programs, he noted that weaknesses in pre-planning can be overcome by a capacity for embracing error, learning with people, and building and institutionalizing new knowledge through action.

By retaining many of its original staff, BRAC has been fortunate to maintain a strong sense of institutional knowledge. However, now approaching its 40-year anniversary, BRAC has seen many early members move to other institutions, or in some cases, pass away. Creating systems for ensuring individual knowledge feeds into a more systematic process of codifying and maintaining lessons learned is important for BRAC to maintain its ability to constantly evolve.

Knowledge management

The Research and Evaluation Division (RED) provides external monitoring of program quality. It investigates areas of great programmatic significance that cannot be understood through routine data alone. For example, over the years, RED has investigated the reasons behind *shebika* dropout and gender disparities in delays in accessing TB treatment. In 2011, RED presented data on how incidence rates of TB in *shebikas* compared to the general population. Issues of infection control were raised and implications for program

> "We have seen that the challenge for BRAC is to have a system by which you are able to learn, and learn not only the positive things but the failures, the challenges. In BRAC that's done in many different levels: obviously on the frontline, you learn on a daily basis. The challenge though is, how do you build a system by which you know that the front-line workers are having problems?"
>
> *Mushtaque Chowdhury, Rockefeller Foundation, formerly BRAC*

protocols are now topics of discussion within the department. Concurrently several other projects were underway, with topics including nutritional status and TB, DOTS in hard-to-reach areas and a knowledge, attitudes, and practices (KAP) survey of TB. As BRAC considers refinements to its delivery model, RED brings to bear a wealth of analytical expertise and capability to inform the dialog. Over the years, many staff members have transitioned from RED to the health program, or vice versa, creating an even deeper understanding of the synergies these two departments can achieve.

9.8 Finances and accounting

In 2010, Bangladesh came in 134 out of 178 countries in Transparency International's corruption perception index (TI, 2010). "In the Bangladeshi context, it just doesn't work to have the same manager making all the program decisions and supervising the finances. Misappropriation just happens too often" says Shib Narayan Kairy, the BRAC Group Chief Financial Officer. BRAC has invested tremendously in creating a strong image of financial accountability. It has a central finance and accounts office that handles these activities for all departments. Currently, the office handles all transactions, or approximately US $412 million each year, including US $141 million from donors. All funds for BRAC's international programs are also managed by the Bangladesh office. Maintaining the funds with adequate documentation and systems is critical for maintaining donor trust and program performance. Each donor has its own restrictions on how funds can be spent and what reporting they require. The finance department manages these regulations and works with the program staff to ensure that the criteria are constantly upheld. They value a transparent system and strive to be forthcoming in sharing financial information. All directors get a monthly report on their program's financial activities, and the chief financial officer receives all of them.

With Bangladesh's successful bids for the Global Fund, since 2004 BRAC has had the additional responsibility of sub-contracting to other NGOs and monitoring their activities. This is also handled by the finance and accounting office in communication with the health program staff. BRAC monitors and supervises the finances of these NGOs with the same strict codes of zero tolerance for corruption it holds for its own offices. Financial irregularities are investigated and depending on the nature of the situation, funding can be postponed or terminated.

For BRAC's health program, much of the spending occurs at the local level. Each branch office has its own bank account, and money is transferred to these accounts for staff salaries, incidental expenses, and other program needs. All expenses are also recorded locally, by project, and sent to the head office. BRAC migrated to an electronic accounting system at the branch office level in 2004. However, moving away from paper at the local level poses difficulties as many offices still lack a reliable supply of electricity and have no internet connectivity. Currently, BRAC collects the monthly data by CD. A web-based system would enable much more rapid reporting and real-time analysis, but the infrastructural challenges to implementing it remain great.

Despite these challenges, BRAC's system runs relatively smoothly. Kairy boasts that BRAC has paid all staff on time for the entire 29 years that he's been with the department. Efficient finances are a prerequisite to good implementation; the health program benefits greatly from its ability to rely on a strong accounting department. With 80 central office staff, and 6,000 in local branch offices, it is an extensive team. While some staff work with all programs, many programs also have dedicated staff who exclusively support their activities. The TB program has five staff at the central level. As part of their work, they are expected to know the TB program staff and, in addition, the TB program itself. "They have to know what the TB program is doing to do their job. I always tell my staff, 'please learn the program, please go and see the program, see what they are doing. You can't prioritize your work otherwise.' If the accountants don't know, it's difficult to make good decisions, and it's not a good way to run the program," explains Kairy. Processes for proposal writing are similarly collaborative, with the project and finance staff co-developing budget proposals. For high-level decisions, program directors discuss their plans with the director of finance to ensure alignment between any plans and limitations on the use of the funds.

BRAC's scale enables it to have a dedicated finance and accounts department with extensive capacity to support programs. Many other NGOs are unable to replicate these operations. However, the basic principles of creating some separation between finance and program management and systems for accountability are universally applicable. Furthermore, for NGOs that are interested in scaling up their activities, investments in accounting and development of a multi-level system will be critical. While the independence between BRAC's finance and health program is valuable, the close collaboration allows them to combine forces to perform tasks as efficiently as possible. As evidenced from BRAC's experience, there are few substitutes for good inter-departmental communication.

9.9 Checks and balances

With a budget of close to US $412 million and 47,000 full-time staff, no individual can account for all activities and financial transactions (BRAC, 2011). BRAC must be vigilant in maintaining the organization's reputation and integrity. BRAC was first motivated to create a monitoring unit in 1980, when it implemented performance-based incentives for its Oral Therapy Extension Program and needed a group to conduct follow-up evaluations at the household level test mothers' ability to recreate the solution. In 1990, it created a new unit, independent from both the program and the research and evaluation division, to provide these functions to all programs.

Program monitoring

In addition to each program's own internal data collection activities, the monitoring department collects information on all programs as an external validation mechanism. To ensure that its activities align with the program's priorities, it holds an annual meeting with a group of program staff from all levels to create a list of indicators that will drive monitoring activities for that year. In 2010, areas of interest for the health program included: assessment of antenatal care coverage, incidence of low birthrate in deliveries, and outcomes of patients treated for TB and malaria. The monitoring department collects data based on this list in 2-3% of the program area with its own field monitors (separate from the program staff). Field monitors compile the data and send it to the central office for processing and analysis. The monitoring department staff organize bi-monthly meetings to update to the program staff at the headquarters level on its activities. Once all data are collected, analyzed, and presented to the program staff, the monitoring department prepares a narrative report for the program. In addition, they prepare a one-page report that highlights major findings and areas for required action that is sent to the program and the executive leadership. Six months later, they measure the same indicators and send a follow up report assessing the level of change that has occurred. If no improvement is seen during this period, the executive director may meet with the program director to discuss the issues.

The monitoring department aims to create a participatory process to best enable the programs to understand and utilize its findings. It has found that when the program doesn't feel like a stakeholder in the process, the feedback is largely ignored. They continue to explore methods to increase joint ownership, such as including field staff in the data collection process. However, the value of the monitoring is its neutrality. "Even in the most professional, honest organizations in the world, the MIS data is always inflated. The manager who's running the program is the one looking at the results and making the report. We're there to help, but we just provide the information, programs have to rectify the issues themselves. We want to get the program more involved in the process so that they value the feedback more, but it's critical that we maintain the quality and the neutrality of the process," says Sukhendra K. Sarkar, Director of BRAC's Department of Administration and Risk Management.

Internal audits

The internal audit department scrutinizes program finances from the central level down to every branch office. They concentrate on the microfinance program, given the disproportionate number of financial transactions that place relative to the health and education program. In particular, the program watches to identify instances of misappropriation or other types of irregularities. All staff that work on financial monitoring are based in the central office; they go to the field to conduct interviews and examine the account books.

When suspicious activity is found, the auditor writes a report that is sent to the location of the activity and the program director. The program is expected to submit a response within 30 days explaining the situation and outlining its planned actions of remedy. Often upon review, an accounting error is identified that explains the difference. Based on the response, the auditor either closes the case, or convenes the audit review committee that is composed of a few other directors.

For the most extreme cases, a special audit review committee with two governing board members can be convened. The outcome of the case depends on the nature of the explanations, the information, and implementation of recommendations. "BRAC has a zero tolerance policy on corruption. It doesn't matter if one taka or one crore taka was misappropriated. We treat it the same way," Sarkar emphasizes.

In financial auditing as with program monitoring, the department faces the same struggle about how to integrate the program into the process sufficiently to enable change, but without compromising the neutrality. The greatest obstacle likely is the existing burden on the program directors. Sarkar comments, "They are so overloaded with their program responsibilities, they don't have time to look at the data and analyze it. And if you don't analyze it, what good is it? In theory you should be able to use the MIS data to flag some of the issues. Having sensors inside the program and outside the program would be ideal."

These are issues that all programs struggle with—the external lens promotes neutrality and independent assessment, which are healthy to program growth and quality. However, complete separation increases the investment necessary to integrate the results and feedback into program activities. Finding a balance is an ongoing process between departments.

9.10 Staying nimble

> "Separation [of those with day-to-day contact with the community reality and those with decision-making roles] is not found in the success cases examined...the process of rapid, creative adaptation essential for achieving and sustaining the fit on which effective performance depends nearly demands such integration."
>
> *David Korten (Korten, 1980)*

In BRAC's early years, there was no division between operations and top-level decision making; the team was small enough that those overseeing field activities were also engaged in the central planning meetings. As BRAC has grown over the years, it has had to find ways to protect its core skill of ensuring that feedback from the frontline works its way up to the ears of BRAC's leaders. In addition to strong mechanisms for routine data collection and frequent field visits by middle-level staff, much of the feedback is still communicated verbally. Mushtaque comments that weekly meetings between program managers are a major form of coordination and the basis of operational evolution. "So the weekly meetings help a lot. That's one of the innovations of BRAC, those meetings where they try to resolve issues. Even in the scaled up programs, you need to keep that culture going in order to learn and take actions."

In addition to keeping in step with the changes in the field, BRAC's leadership must scan the horizon more broadly for emerging opportunities. Disciplined foresight has allowed them to keep their edge over time and ensure that BRAC can compete for leadership or new funding as it becomes available. For example, BRAC predicted that education would become a major international priority in the 1990s and as a result began to invest in creating educational programs in the mid-1980s. By the time the donor community mobilized support for universal access to basic education in 1990, BRAC already had a rich portfolio of education programs and was poised to scale with the newly available resources. Abed comments, "In development you really see that luck favors the prepared. To be successful and take programs to scale, you have to develop the practical know-how before the obvious opportunity emerges and you take it up."

What's next in health

Already, there are rumbles of some emerging new priorities in global health, and BRAC must begin to prepare if it wants to have an edge. At the World Health Assembly in May 2011, non-communicable diseases were recognized as one of "the greatest challenges to health and development today." Preparations for a high-level meeting are underway to bring the issue in front of the United Nations General Assembly in September 2011 (WHO, 2011).

Building on its success in providing eye exams and reading glasses at the community level, BRAC is also exploring the feasibility of providing other forms of eye care, such as cataract surgery. However, BRAC is reluctant to move beyond the pilot phase of these activities unless it identifies likely sources of funding for the scale up and sustaining of these programs.

Another area of significant interest in global health is the application of mobile technology to global health. While the concept of telemedicine has been explored for decades, proponents of "mHealth" see it as a tool that could fundamentally transform delivery in resource-limited settings. With the right system, it can enable better disease management, field worker workflow and supervision, data collection and reporting, and many other processes. While certainly there are exciting possibilities on how mHealth could improve service delivery, an organization like BRAC, facing immense costs of changing its current system to a mobile-based one, will tread carefully without demonstrated evidence that the transition is warranted.

Three stages of the learning process

Learning to be effective. Creating a fit between the program model and the beneficiaries' needs. This stage is relatively resource intensive and ideally includes a good deal of intellectual input and experimental latitude. Capacity building, process documentation, and continuous action research should be program priorities. What is required to achieve fit for a given time and setting?

Learning to be efficient. The priority is to reduce the input required per unit to achieve the desired outcome. Important activities are routinized and extraneous activities are eliminated. Some gains of efficiency may come from moving up the learning curve, but efforts to improve efficiency may also compromise the initial effectiveness seen in the first phase. Questions of fit now center on aligning program requirements with realistically attainable organizational capacities.

Learning to expand. Emphasizing expansion of organizational capacity, the focus is on continually ensuring an acceptable level of program fit and weighing trade-offs of efficiency and quality. Rate of growth is largely determined by how much time and resources are required to develop the necessary additional organizational capacities. Once expansion is completed, many organizations turn their attention to tackling new issues in the community.

Korten, 1980

On a small scale, BRAC is piloting a mHealth technology in its urban maternal, neonatal, and child health program, Manoshi. With a group called mPower, Manoshi has a "proof of concept" pilot underway to examine how an mHealth application called "BRAC health" impacts their delivery model. The software guides *shasthya kormis* through a series of questions during a screening with a pregnant woman that determines the level of risk and intensity of support required. Physicians in BRAC's headquarters also receive the patient profiles, enabling them to identify high-risk pregnancies and provide addition follow up. The program organizer can organize the *shasthya kormi's* time, send it to her phone, and then monitor her activities to ensure that she follows it. Currently the project is in intense learning mode; all levels of staff are still getting up to speed on the technology and how to best integrate it into staff workflow. Once the technology has been adequately refined on a small scale, BRAC plans to scale it up across its maternal, neonatal, and child health programs and will look for other opportunities to expand usage of mhealth in its essential health care programming more broadly.

9.11 Managing the external context

Overall, BRAC's own revenue accounts for 70% of its total budget (BRAC, 2010). However, for the health program, almost all funds come from outside donors. Maintaining a positive image and good relationships with other stakeholders is critical to long-term sustainability. The most important relationships are those with the government, other NGOs, and donors.

BRAC respects and supports the government's role in driving the health priorities and policies for Bangladesh, particularly in respect to education and health. As much as possible, it supports the public sector activities in these areas. However, its greatest value add is in its service delivery infrastructure. Therefore, it seeks opportunities to complement public sector activities at the implementation level.

Leaders at BRAC believe strongly that BRAC must work with the government. However, they acknowledge that making partnerships effective is challenging for both parties. At times, the partnership model creates delays in moving from planning to action. Sometimes, BRAC faces bureaucratic hurdles that would not exist if it were working independently. Historically

> In addition to its primary functions of policy, finance, regulation, and implementation, the Ministry of Health and Family Welfare has to take a stewardship role. It brings partners together to design policy, develop strategy, and of course when looking at implementation, it should use the comparative advantage of all stakeholders, public and private. There is plenty of evidence that when we work jointly, we produce greater results. This is true not just for TB, but also for programs like family planning, malaria and maternal and child health.
>
> *Faruque Ahmed, BRAC*

Bangladesh's government has had a positive relationship with NGOs. Since independence, on the whole, Bangladeshis have been extremely optimistic about the country's prospects and growth. Early on, the government realized that it would not be able to realize these expectations by working alone, and invited the country's NGOs to partner with it. As a result, though there are challenges, the environment for public-private partnerships is relatively open and NGOs contribute significantly to public sector activities.

Particularly in recent years, BRAC has begun to work in partnerships with many other organizations and programs within the public sector. These relationships enable more comprehensive service delivery systems, but also create an organized platform for advocacy and joint planning. NGOs can work together to influence political commitment and policy development. BRAC's experiences in the public-private partnership, discussed in Chapter 5, provide more detail on one partnership's experiences in these areas. One lesson that BRAC has learned is that transparent communication is critical to creating the necessary trust. "The worst thing you can do is say one thing to one partner and then turn around and say something else to another. We have to make sure that we're consistent in what we say," Faruque said.

As BRAC expands internationally, it finds itself in new contexts where it must learn to navigate a new political system. *The Economist* reflected, "Its expansion overseas may, however, present BRAC with a new problem. Robert Kaplan, an American writer, says that NGOs fill the void between thousands of villages and a remote, often broken, government. BRAC does this triumphantly in Bangladesh— but it is a Bangladeshi organization. Whether it can do the same elsewhere remains to be seen (*The Economist*, 2010)."

Donor relations

Like most development organizations, BRAC's health program is heavily reliant on the contributions of donors. Though grants account for under a third of BRAC's overall annual expenditure, in the health program, donor funds account for over 90% of the US $32 million budget.

For the most part, donor priorities are well aligned with Bangladesh's health needs. The magnitude of the mortality and

> "Apart from the quality of work on the ground, their attention to detail in concern to the contractual agreements... BRAC really stood out among the grantees I've worked with. In terms of the monitoring visits, everything laid out in the contracts; reporting requirements, requests for additional information; standout in their role as a grantee; importantly I was struck by their concern with how things were going; at the end of every visit, we'd meet with Faruque, and you could tell he was quite serious about the findings, both positive and negative. If anything was not running as it should, he was quite concerned about getting to the bottom of it immediately, not down the road. Similarly any recommendations we made, by the next month or next visit they'd be carefully considered at the very least. It is unusual, based on our experiences, for a grantee to take so seriously the findings."
>
> I.D. Rusen, *International Union against Tuberculosis and Lung Disease*

morbidity related to malaria and TB, and high rates of mortality in mothers, infants and children merit their own programs within BRAC's health portfolio. Several insiders and outsiders comment that there has been increasing verticalization of BRAC's programs at least at the management level because of the segregated funding streams. However, as the *shebika* represents the frontline worker for the majority of programs, it is difficult to argue that these changes have had implications that reach the delivery model.

Media and communications

In today's era of globalization, an organization of BRAC's size needs a focused communications strategy. Creating a reputation of transparency, financial accountability, and program success is critical to satisfying current donors, influencing policy-makers, and creating opportunities for new partnerships. New forms of media and networking enable faster sharing of information—BRAC can share the successes of its approaches and learn from other implementers real-time.

In 2007, BRAC's achievements in TB were recognized at annual conference of the International Union against TB and Lung Disease, where BRAC was one of two winners of the prestigious Stop TB Partnership-Kochon Prize (Stop TB, 2011). The award, which includes a prize of US $65,000, highlights an individual and organizations that for "extraordinary contributions to fighting TB."

BRAC received the award "for scaling up TB control in Bangladesh by involving communities and increasing access to diagnosis and treatment."

International interest in BRAC's TB program led to additional opportunities to disseminate its experiences. The *New York Times* featured an article about BRAC's shebikas and the bond system (Sengupta, 2007). In 2007, BRAC was approached by faculty at Harvard University about developing a case study on its TB program. These opportunities enable BRAC to gain international recognition for its community approaches and strengthen BRAC's "brand." The brand enables BRAC to gain the trust of new partners, particularly in its international work and to participate in policy dialog at the global level. BRAC can also leverage this reputation and track record when approaching donors with innovative ideas that push the bounds of scientific knowledge or public health norms.

In addition to media exposure, targeting leaders in advanced economies that control resources for international development is important to ensure continuity of support. BRAC has also partnered with RESULTS, an international advocacy group that supports increasing resources to address poverty and create access to health care. Its executive director, Joanne Carter, accompanied several US senators and helped organize a congressional delegation educational trip to visit Bangladesh to see firsthand the impact that Global Fund resources enabled. In addition, RESULTS has facilitated the visits of British and Canadian members of parliament, creating opportunities for them to observe BRAC's TB programs at the community level and how grants are utilized to reach poor TB patients.

9.12 Sustainability

When Abed founded BRAC, he expected it to become obsolete in just a few years' time. And yet, BRAC has only continued to expand and become increasingly entrenched in health and development efforts in Bangladesh. Its health and development programs, especially those targeting the poor and ultra-poor, are still largely reliant on donor funds. Given the fragility of available resources and the constant changes in global priorities, how does BRAC think about issues of sustainability? Is there a day when Bangladesh will no longer need a BRAC?

BRAC considers sustainability at every level of program design. It considers the implications for field level activities if the program support ceased overnight. The beauty of the volunteer model is that *shebikas* would maintain their knowledge, and many would likely find ways to continue receiving payments for their services. Constant efforts to invest in public sector capacity and ownership also contribute to a sense that BRAC's efforts support the creation of a permanent backbone and health infrastructure.

However, BRAC's leaders now see the problems of poverty, lack of education and poor health as problems that will require decades to truly overcome. While government capacity is increasing, it is unlikely that in the next 10-20 years they will develop enough to absorb the current efforts of NGOs, of which BRAC is one of the largest contributors. Imran Matin, deputy executive director of BRAC's international program, comments that poverty eradication requires a 50-year timeframe. Therefore, BRAC will need to continue investing in relationships with donors and advocacy at the global level to sustain availability of funds for its programming.

9.13 International expansion

As discussed in Chapter 8, BRAC first established programs outside of Bangladesh in 2002, when it expanded to Afghanistan. In 2005, the devastating tsunami in Sri Lanka created another moment when BRAC felt compelled to provide post-disaster rehabilitation and livelihood regeneration efforts. In subsequent years, BRAC has expanded its health programs to Pakistan, Haiti, and five countries in Africa: Uganda, Tanzania, Southern Sudan, Liberia, and Sierra Leone.

Imran Matin moved from director of RED to serve as the deputy in the newly formed international program in 2005, directed by Aminul Alam. BRAC initially conceived the unit as one of its programs, but the complexity of delivering a set of programs in a range of international contexts proved to be a much greater undertaking that required more comprehensive support than any other single program. Also, because of regulatory restrictions on moving money out of Bangladesh, new financial practices were required for the international programs. In 2008, BRAC registered as a charity in the Netherlands to provide greater financial flexibility and transparency, an important requirement for attracting donors.

In early 2005, BRAC began to explore the possibilities of moving to Africa, particularly Anglophone countries. BRAC also sought governments that were supportive of their activities; in Uganda, for example, first lady Janet Museveni came to visit the Bangladesh programs herself in 2005. When visiting potential countries, BRAC also assessed a country's readiness for microfinance and the availability of these services. In Kenya, for example, a country were BRAC ultimately decided not to work, BRAC saw huge amounts of microfinance programs already running and felt that its impact would be minimal. BRAC felt there was potential for it to provide large-scale development programs in Uganda and Tanzania, and in 2006, initiated microfinance, health and agriculture programs. Southern Sudan was a country that it prioritized based on the tremendous need, but BRAC felt that getting a bit of footing in East Africa prior to entering would allow it to operate more effectively. In 2007, it began programs there.

Thirty years after its early experiences with village organizations, BRAC still found microfinance to provide a sturdy platform for its other programs. "Our strategy was to start with a program that could be lifted from Bangladesh and adapted locally. It was a way to get the ball rolling and we could adapt as we learned. Microfinance was the easiest from that standpoint. It involves intensive interaction with the community, which provides a lot of opportunity to learn. It also has very concrete and quantifiable metrics, which is really important when you're working with new staff and just getting started. It also can be scaled quickly and in a way that facilitates the addition of other programs," Imran reflected.

BRAC as an organization is still learning how to operate internationally and leverage its reach most effectively. While to date, learning has been predominantly unilateral, as the international programs mature and develop the capacity to innovate locally, in the future there will be opportunities for Bangladesh to learn from its other programs. In several countries, microfinance will require BRAC to become a regulated entity, and it will need to confront questions of deposit taking, standardization or tier-levels of branches, and other implications. Imran notes, "Right now, we're facing a host of very tricky but relevant operational issues that we'll eventually have to sort out here. It just so happens that we'll have to confront them first in Africa, and when we get to that stage in Bangladesh, we'll be able to learn from our experiences there."

The same questions that BRAC faces at the program level, around decentralization, communication, management, and capacity building, all apply at the country level as well. There are many opportunities to leverage across countries and departments, but only if the systems and strategies are in place to facilitate them. Leadership at BRAC continues to assess the organization's ability to grow effectively and tries to identify areas for improvement in structure or processes.

Strategy and scale

Just as strategic fit determines the sustainability of profit in the private sector, so too does it drive a development organization's ability to sustain impact. As small organizations demonstrate success and find opportunities to scale, they often dilute the original value proposition by expanding into areas where they lack expertise and capabilities or make compromises to the activity system. To scale effectively, an organization must find ways to *deepen* its strategic positioning through growth.

BRAC focuses on low intensity programs that require deep community knowledge but not high levels of technical expertise or clinical specialization. They look for opportunities to tackle common health conditions with relatively standard interventions, rather than rare conditions or ones that require significant customization of services.

In international expansion, BRAC has recognized that post-conflict countries represent locations where it can have a significant impact. It focuses on the rural populations in these countries, as even in Bangladesh it is still learning the dynamics of the complex urban environment.

9.14 Conclusions

BRAC offers a glimpse at a mature NGO that has forty years of investment and experience. The balance between preserving those qualities that made BRAC effective, such as its willingness to listen to communities and respond dynamically to new observations, and creating a strong operational apparatus that's crucial for large-scale programming is an ongoing challenge. Institutionalization creates sustainability, but threatens entrepreneurial behavior and operational agility. BRAC tries to minimize these effects by allowing the programs to focus on programming and move the administrative and financial issues to other units. However, close department collaboration requires investments that are not always organic. BRAC has an international reputation for its accountability and sound financial practices, yet within the programs, leaders continue to think about how these can be improved and further integrated into the programs themselves. Health information technology and trends like mHealth demonstrate the increasing number of tools that programs have to choose from and the potential for increasing transparency, accountability, ability to make data-informed decision making, and efficiency at every level.

BRAC challenges the conventional notion of what a "sustainable" program entails. As a homegrown organization, it draws on and contributes to human resource capacity in Bangladesh. Its overhead costs are relatively low, and it has become increasingly financially self-sufficient over the years. BRAC's partnerships with the public sector have weathered several changes in administration, and despite increasing capacity in the health system, it is unlikely that the need for BRAC's support will diminish anytime soon.

Maintaining program relevance in a quickly changing environment is a challenge for any organization, but particularly one implementing a standardized model to millions. BRAC's ability to evolve will be tested by rapid changes in technology, urbanization, and shifts in epidemiology. Its history demonstrates adaptability and foresight in predicting trends, and it must continue to protect and strengthen these abilities to survive.

While at scale already, as its international programs grow, BRAC will be forced to re-confront these questions of integration vs. specialization within its organizational structure. BRAC's international programs rely on the Bangladesh headquarters for many of these processes, which may impede their local growth or effectiveness.

BRAC's mission and sense of global responsibility continues to grow. While programming is its instinctive preference, it possesses a wealth of knowledge that could benefit other implementers and policy-makers. By disseminating and sharing its expertise with others, it can have a much larger potential impact than it could achieve operating alone.

Chapter 10

Beyond TB: Potential Applications

"Medicines don't work if you don't take them."
Surgeon General Everett Koop

BRAC designed its model for the specific characteristics of TB in rural Bangladesh in the 1980s. In the last 27 years, much has changed globally—in the epidemiological burden, in our understanding of health and disease, and in the resources available in developing countries for health. We see many opportunities to apply what we've learned to the health issues that face Bangladesh and other developing countries worldwide. The thoughts here are mainly exploratory, motivated by our belief that the large-scale delivery of health interventions, especially involving long-term care, is one of the most urgent challenges in global health. We will discuss the relevance BRAC's TB control model to other conditions demonstrate potential areas of broader application.[1]

10.1 Distilling a transferable framework from BRAC's TB delivery model

BRAC's particular success has been in creating a model and management system that's conducive to scale and realistic in its requirements (financial and otherwise) for lower-middle incomes settings. For governments and others interested in achieving scale in their efforts to provide long-term care at the community-level, BRAC's experience and reflections will be particularly useful in developing local implementation strategies.

---

[1] We use the term "*shebika*" instead of the generic term "volunteer" to refer to the specific hybrid model of incentives, support, and supervision that BRAC's model in Bangladesh includes. This model is discussed in depth in Chapter 6.

What makes the model work?

Based on its experience with refining the model for TB care, BRAC has noted some characteristics that were critical for its effectiveness. BRAC's initial model aimed to achieve these capabilities in the context of rural Bangladesh; as it expands into new contexts and as Bangladesh itself changes, the model must update to preserve these characteristics through new activities. We will briefly list them here as these are discussed in depth in Chapters 2, 6, and the Conclusion.

- **Competence and character of frontline staff.** A *shebika* must be technically qualified for her responsibilities, but it is equally important that she garners trust from the community and individuals.

- **Patient experience and participation.** BRAC's management and operations system is designed so as to maintain the range of programs at large scale. The patient's experience is simple as there is one person per village who serves to provide access to all health services and products. A key component of BRAC's model is the active engagement of the patient in the treatment process as the patient and provider sign a bond agreement to complete therapy.

- **Intensive supervision and support.** Supervision is a key component of the management system as both the program officer and *shasthya kormi* (health worker) provide supervision and problem solving. These activities create a standard of quality and ensure that *shebika* does not feel alone in her responsibilities.

- **Part of a larger package.** BRAC's TB program is integrated into a larger package of goods and services provided by the *shebika*. These other activities create additional visibility, and demand for her services, giving her more opportunities to actively screen for TB symptoms and meet other health needs of her community. It also creates an element of trust in her work and commitment.

These components are synergistic. BRAC has created a systematic process to identify individuals who are likely to be effective as *shebikas*. It is the combination of the right person *and* the right management that create an effective model. In addition, the bond creates an investment on the part of the patient so that the patients are motivated to share transfers, moves, treatment concerns, and other issues with their provider. When patients transfer or experience side effects that require additional treatment, they inform the *shebika* so that they are eligible to receive their bond. As the *shebika* is in close proximity, it's easy to inform her. If the patient misses a dose of treatment, the *shebika* knows that day. She can also alert her superiors if more complex care is indicated.

10.2 Application to other medical conditions

Non-adherence is a universal issue in conditions requiring an extended course of treatment, first identified in the literature over 60 years ago (Chesney, 2006). It is a concern on two levels: first, a patient incompletely treated may not be cured, and second, in the treatment of microbial infections can lead to drug resistance and lead to infections in others that are more difficult to treat. It's estimated that one half of patients do not receive the full benefit from their treatment because of non-adherence. Clearly, creating models that raise rates of adherence is essential in improving health worldwide (Chesney, 2006). In contrast, BRAC treated close to 96,000 patients for TB in 2009. Of these, only 1,311 defaulted, a rate of approximately 1.4%. All other patients were accounted for by the program, and over 90% were cured. As BRAC has demonstrated that a disease requiring a daily regimen for six months can be effectively treated at the community level and managed at scale, we consider whether this model could be adapted for HIV/AIDS or non-communicable disease.

The place to begin is with the *shebikas*. What types of services are they capable of performing? How much training will be necessary to make them effective diagnosticians and therapists? Below is a diagram of what activities in the care delivery value chain for tuberculosis can be performed by a *shebika* in a community, and which steps require engagement of higher-level staff or facility-based care. For tuberculosis, almost all activities can be performed at the community level, except in the case of complex diagnosis, side effects, or drug resistance. These are handled in BRAC's system primarily through referrals to other providers that have these capabilities.

The majority of required activities can be performed by the community health worker (Table 10.1). In addition, she can facilitate the activities that require other health providers by linking them with the patient. The medical officer is necessary to make the diagnosis and as a referral for side effects, but much of TB care has been set in protocols that do not require medical expertise for daily treatment. In addition, the *shebika's* proximity and ability to provide social support in the community context can have additional benefits for a disease like TB where stigma may be an issue.

Table 10.1: Adapted care delivery value chain for tuberculosis[2]

Required skill level	Stage				
	Broad prevention	Screening	Diagnosis	Management	Follow-up
Can be performed by *shebika*	Education, Stigma reduction	Household visits, Inquiring about symptoms	Assistance in sputum collection, Accompaniment to sputum smearing sites	DOTS treatment, Collecting sputum for follow-up checks	Vigilance about return of symptoms
Performed in the community by higher-trained provider			Staffing of sputum smearing outreach sites	Management of side effects	
Requires facility-based care			Diagnosis of sputum smear negative, extra-pulmonary, drug resistant TB	Management of serious side effects	Drug resistance testing if indicated

We will explore whether the model has a similar application for other chronic conditions, such as HIV/AIDS and hypertension, to compare how well the required activities might match the *shebikas'* capabilities. In these examples, the duration of support is much longer what TB requires. In many ways, this increases the importance of a contract explicitly outlining the dual responsibility of the provider and the patient. However, it does raise questions of how to design the incentive component, whether it is a monetary payment, a public award, or an item of value (e.g. blanket or bicycle), so that it

---

[2] The care delivery value chain was designed by Porter and Teisberg, 2006. What is presented here is a modified version that draws on some of its key concepts.

maintains the incentives indefinitely. Supervising adherence to a medical regimen is perhaps simpler than supervising behavioral changes; how to incorporate support for non-medical treatments is another area of inquiry that these applications will require.

10.3 HIV/AIDS

Since the early 1980s, HIV has changed the face of health worldwide, particularly in sub-Saharan Africa. Scientific advances and resource mobilization have expanded the availability of treatment in the last decade. Globally, deaths from HIV dropped by 20% from 2004 to 2009, primarily because of the rapid expansion of antiretroviral therapy (ART) (MSF, 2011). This dramatic decline was enabled by dedicated commitment for what was framed as a "global emergency;" vertical treatment programs were scaled quickly largely outside of the existing health systems, which were deemed too fragile or weak to withstand the desired speed of rollout. No longer a death sentence in developing countries, HIV is increasingly a chronic condition that requires ongoing management and access to other health services, programs must transition to an "integrated and durable approach" anchored in the health system (Atun and Bataringaya, 2011). Implementers must adopt a paradigm shift that recognizes the need to management systems capable of supporting large cohorts of patients on ART and expanding access to those who currently lack treatment.

Updating programs should include emphasis on improving patient adherence and retention. Adherence to ART strongly predicts viral suppression, drug resistance, disease progression, and death (Bangsberg and Deeks, 2010). By prevent drug resistance (which requires switching to second-line drugs), it also reduces treatment costs. An annual supply of the WHO-recommended first-line daily medication for one patient can be purchased in many countries for around US $180. Second-line treatment is at least three times this amount (MSF, 2011). The cumulative burden of these costs is staggering; reducing and delaying the failure of first-line drugs significantly lowers a program's pharmaceutical costs, allowing more patients to be treated with a given amount of resources.

Many epidemiologists, program implementers and others advocate for global mobilization to initiate antiretroviral treatment much earlier (raising the threshold from current guidelines around

CD4 count and other criteria). This is motivated by a range of scientific and economic reasons, including evidence that it would yield: decreased transmission of the virus; improved clinical outcomes; cost effectiveness in reducing mortality, illness and hospitalization, and prevention of opportunistic infections, like TB, that also pose public health concerns (MSF, 2011). "Treatment as prevention" has been recently demonstrated to reduce the likelihood of transmission to others, including regular partners and spouses (Donnell et al., 2010). Mechanisms to motivate high levels of adherence and identification of potential beneficiaries are crucial assumptions in the population-level benefits that this is projected to generate.

Non-adherence, however, remains one of the common challenges to HIV programs and has the potential to undermine any strategy to scale up access. A high "lost-to-follow up" (LTFU) rate, a term coined to measure the percentage of patients that are not known to be dead or receiving care elsewhere and have no contact with the clinic (or pharmacy) for three months or more, obscures thorough examination of a delivery model's achievements of adherence. Programs with high LTFU rates may present misleadingly positive patient outcomes, as often it is the sicker patients that fail to return for treatment (Losina et al., 2009). In one study looking at 15 sites across Asia, Africa and South America, the average LTFU rate was 20% for the first six months of ART treatment (Brinkof et al., 2008). Another review found that at two years, an average of 60% of ART patients in Africa are retained by programs (Rosen et al., 2007). Comparative studies find that active follow up reduces the number of patients lost, but as programs scale, they often abandon this activity. It is estimated that in resource-limited settings, approximately 50% of those LTFU are dead (Brinkof et al., 2008). For these reasons, the rate of retention and the proportion of patients remaining alive and on ART (at a designated point in time) are gaining acceptance as a litmus test of program performance and evidence of long-term success (Atun and Bataringaya, 2011).

Community-based adherence models offer an opportunity to counteract some of these trends. Qualitative research on HIV indicates that for many patients, the challenges with adherence are not limited to simply taking the medication; many struggle with the psychological coping process that the lifelong disease requires. In communities where HIV carries stigma, patients may be reluctant to disclose their illness and then consequently suffer from social isolation and discrimination related to their status (Obermeyer, Baijal, Pegurri, 2011). There is significant empirical evidence that community-based DOTS can be implemented effectively (Bangsberg and Deeks, 2010). Some of these programs have argued that community-based programming can reduce stigma while providing critical social support at a close proximity (Behforouz, Farmer, Mukherjee, 2004).

As programs have matured and transitioned from an emergency mode to a health system strengthening mode, there has been an increase in efforts to decentralize HIV care, physically as well as in the delivery models. In public and private HIV programs alike, evidence for community-based care has motivated significant task-shifting and an embrace of community health workers and lay counselors to provide HIV testing and adherence support (MSF, 2011). In addition to relieving some burden on health facilities, research demonstrates that community-based care relieves patients of costs associated with treatment, such as transportation, lost earnings, and time (Bangsberg and Deeks, 2010). Advocates of this approach are quick to warn that without attention to training, supervision and other management issues, these programs will not provide quality support, thus failing to produce the desired increases in retention of care and reduction in lost-to-follow-up rates (Hermann et al., 2009, 31).

Applying the BRAC TB model

Many of the activities involved in HIV care can be performed by a *shebika*. Increasingly, HIV testing is being performed in non-clinical settings. Rapid diagnostics have enabled programs to launch home-based testing programs and send counselors into communities to provide testing. Linking these patients with care and support is critical if these activities are to result in reductions in mortality and morbidity.

Non-adherence has emerged as a problem for programs globally, in both high and low income countries. Community-based solutions can effectively address many of the diffuse causes for skipping doses by: providing frequent reminders to take medicines; insuring that patients understand their treatment; reducing financial constraints; and providing a regular supply of drugs (Mills et al., 2006). Side effects are a common cause of dropout but could be reduced by early identification and on the spot referrals and linkages to care. Though the issue of stigmatization is often raised as a factor that limits community-based care, this has not been the experience of the BRAC DOTS program. To the contrary, the open acceptance of illness and the clear demonstration that care is being provided may actually reduce stigmatization. Clearly, for many patients, community-based care has great potential to eliminate many barriers to adherence.

Table 10.2: Adapted care delivery value chain for HIV/AIDS

Required skill level	Stage				
	Broad prevention	Screening	Diagnosis	Management	Follow-up
Can be performed by *shebika*	Education, Stigma reduction, Provision of condoms, clean syringes	Counseling around risk behaviours, symptoms Pregnant mothers	Accompanying patient to testing	DOTS for ARV, Accompaniment to appointments, Referrals, Screening for TB	Psychological support
Performed in the community by higher-trained provider			Rapid HIV testing	Check up with stable patients	
Requires facility-based care			Initial staging	Monitoring of CD4 count and viral load, Management of serious side efforts, Management of opportunistic infections (OI)	Switch to second-line drugs when indicated, Palliative care

From Table 10.2, it's clear that most of the required activities can be performed at the community level by the *shebika*. Many programs already use community health workers or volunteers to oversee treatment and there is ample research demonstrating that this can be an efficacious and cost effective strategy. In considering BRAC's TB model, two areas of particular importance are its active case finding and strong support for adherence. Countries searching for community-based programs to use at scale may find the BRAC model for TB instructive.

One significant difference in HIV and TB is the duration of treatment. Most TB patients complete treatment in six months. HIV infection requires lifelong treatment. Can an investment strategy be developed when treatment will last for many years, perhaps indefinitely? One approach could be to create a rollover contract with the bond that was renewed every 4-6 months at a patient's regular check-up. This could be an interest bearing account with the money accumulating over time. As patients would receive this interest at the time of check-up they would be further motivated to make their appointments, inform the provider of moves or their discontinuing of care, which would drastically reduce the LTFU rate. If they failed to report these changes within a specific period of time and failed to report for treatment, the bond would be forfeited. If the patient died, the family would have to report this to receive the balance of the contract including the original capitation fee. Field testing the intervention would be essential to determine the effectiveness of this approach. Given the endemic challenges of LTFU, particularly in large-scale programs, there is merit to exploring different types of contracts to see what effect they have on patient behavior, provider behavior, and outcomes. It is important to note that the bond is not for payment of drugs or testing but rather to acknowledge the value of community-based care. Patients would retain the option of seeking services with no bond system at the health facilities.

Many are calling for increased operational research and new systems to expand access to services and enhance patient adherence and retention (Atun and Bataringaya, 2011). The BRAC model should be replicated to see how it would work with HIV/AIDS. While the variations and potential designs are numerous, the basic premise would be that there is a bond, put up by the patient, which is returned (or provides regular interest) on continuation of care and forfeited if the patient drops out without informing the provider. Field testing is necessary to assess the applicability of these concepts and how to align the incentives optimally.

10.4 Application to non-communicable disease

Despite the serious challenges that HIV and other infectious diseases present, deaths due to infectious disease are on the global decline and awareness about the burden of disease caused by non-communicable disease is growing. As life expectancy increases in many low and middle-income countries and populations adopt lifestyles lacking physical activity and healthy diets, the burden on non-communicable diseases has burgeoned. Environmental factors, such as indoor smoking and biomass fuel, also contribute to the burden. Cardiovascular disease alone claims 17.4 million lives annually, and 80% of these are in low and middle-income countries (WHO, 2007, 8). From 2006 to 2015, deaths from non-communicable are expected to increase by 17%, with cardiovascular disease accounting for about half of the increase (WHO, 2007, 8).

Risk factors for early onset cardiovascular disease include high blood sugar (diabetes), hypertension, high lipid levels, and tobacco use. These proximal determinants are related to behavioral factors such as poor diet, lack of physical activity and obesity (WHO, 2007, 12). While we will focus on the application to hypertension, prevention or treatment of many other non-communicable diseases could be addressed with similar strategies.

10.5 Hypertension

Hypertension is estimated to cause seven million premature deaths annually (WHO, 2007, 46). Treating it results in a 35-40% reduction of the risk of stroke and 16% reduction in risk of myocardial infarction. It primarily presents in the middle-aged years and is diagnosed with a blood pressure test that can be performed by a nurse or trained health worker using an electronic blood pressure cuff. Given the ease of its diagnosis, often the best screening tactic is to test all people over a certain age threshold and others with a family history or other risk factors. This allows for lifestyle changes and treatment to begin prior to complications or other adverse events.

Reducing salt intake is important for reducing hypertension. Excessive salt intake is seen in many communities and admittedly is a difficult behavior to change. But this is just the kind of intervention that a village-based worker is likely to be able to correct as she observes food preparation and eating habits (Table 10.3). She can also promote physical activity and provide support for smoking cessation, critical lifestyle modifications that can reduce hypertension. Often, daily oral medication is recommended as an additional preventive measure. Given that drug prices can usually be kept low by using generic products, this likely could be a cost effective strategy in developing country settings (WHO, 2003).

Observational studies indicate that conditions like depression, anxiety, lack of social support and isolation all have an independent influence on risk of coronary heart disease. Therefore, daily contact with a care provider from the community may have additional therapeutic benefits that are not yet well quantified by the literature (WHO, 2007, 44-45).

Again, adherence remains the critical challenge to overcome. As many as 40% of patients drop out in the first year of treatment for hypertension, often as a response to side effects of medication (WHO, 2003). Of those that continue, studies indicate that only 50% adhere to their prescribed regimen. As with DOTS, a contract could be developed between the where the patient would agree to take medication and follow certain lifestyle modifications and the provider would periodically check blood pressure, monitor diet, and follow drug adherence. Patients could be rewarded for maintaining a blood pressure that fits a realistic profile and the community-based worker could receive incentives for keeping patients within a certain acceptable range. Studies would have to assess whether adherence increased significantly over baseline.

Table 10.3: Adapted care delivery value chain for hypertension

| Required skill level | Stage | | | | |
	Broad prevention	Screening	Diagnosis	Management	Follow-up
Can be performed by *shebika*	Education on healthy diet, physical activity, tobacco cessation	Target by age, symptoms, BMI if appropriate	Accompanying patient to screening, Blood pressure exam	Encouragement of lifestyle changes, Support for oral treatment	
Performed in the community by higher-trained provider				Regular blood pressure checks, Side effects for medication	
Requires facility-based care				Management of cardiovascular events	

10.6 Conclusions

Here we've focused on describing just two conditions to which BRAC's model for TB treatment could be applied. There are others. Community-based programming creates opportunities for education and behavior modification that prevents disease. It also enables early screenings and timely treatment, with a strong combination of convenience, psychosocial support, and supervision. These components are particularly important for conditions such as chronic obstructive pulmonary disease (COPD), which have a strong environmental component, or issues that require significant behavior modification, such as tobacco cessation. BRAC's experience demonstrates that this model can be implemented at a size sufficient to have an impact on population health and to realize economies of scale.

Another important element to consider in the applicability of this model is how activities related to different conditions could be integrated and synergistic. In some contexts, especially in southern sub-Saharan Africa, co-morbidity of HIV and TB is quite high and programs attempting to address these conditions will need to consider them together. Similarly, the activities required for hypertension prevention and care have significant overlap with those that are required for other conditions, such as diabetes. With additional training, a *shebika* could handle screening and treatment support for both; additional costs would largely be limited to diagnostics and medications. Frameworks such as the one presented here that start at the level of listing the activities, can be useful in determining potential leverage points.

BRAC's TB program has demonstrated that a *shebika* model capable of high levels of case detection, adherence to drugs, and life style changes can be implemented and sustained at scale. Our goal has been to describe a model that's not only effective, but capable of covering a large number of people. In Chapter 9, we discussed the management that program scale up requires. However, the perfect management system will not help patients without an effective delivery model. These lessons will be particularly applicable as programs seek strategies for reducing costs without compromising the effectiveness of their program. Effective programming at the community level has the potential to stretch resources further, allowing more patients to access health care. Community health workers are a powerful provider of psychosocial support and constant supervision, both important determinants of adherence and well being. Agreeing to a contract with the patient before he or she enters treatment solidifies expectations and creates an important sense of mutual responsibility. Programs have the responsibility to first choose the right individuals, then train them effectively, motivate them, monitor and support them, and retain them. Linkages to other providers and more complex types of care are essential for ensuring that their activities yield improved patient outcomes. Combining adherence support with peer support groups may be required for conditions that require greater lifestyle modifications or are currently incurable. Similarly, these variations in disease conditions will require experimentation with the bond system to align incentives effectively and in a way that sustains motivation.

As described in Chapter 6, some medical conditions are more conducive to a community-based model than others. In the case of TB, there was extensive scientific and clinical knowledge about the disease. In addition, there was low diagnostic variability; all patients with TB were clinically indicated to initiate standard treatment. Patients also responded to treatment or did not, and failure was easy to identify (sputum tests during treatment) (Bohmer, 2005). HIV and hypertension have similar characteristics that facilitate application of the *shebika* model.

These characteristics are not static; as clinical knowledge and diagnostics advance, there may be new tools to manage or reduce variability for many chronic diseases. This phenomenon occurred in the diagnosis and treatment of HIV/AIDS, as we've moved from a limited understanding of the clinical progression to thorough guidelines, management strategies, and treatment regimens over the past 30 years. Community health workers could not have treated HIV in the 1990s because it would have been impossible to equip them with the amount of medical decision-making skill necessary to manage the patients responsibly. Fifteen years later, this is standard practice. This is not to say that clinical specialization is becoming obsolete; on the contrary, it can be reserved for the complex cases that need it most.

The TB model provides an example of a scalable, community-based model that effectively produces a high level of patient and provider adherence, challenges which impede many public health efforts worldwide. We believe that these principles should be explored for different diseases in different settings.

Chapter 11

Conclusions: The Luxury of Working in Bangladesh

"The world is moving so fast these days that the man who says it can't be done is generally interrupted by someone doing it."

Elbert Hubbard

BRAC has quietly worked in Bangladesh for the past 40 years. Usually it preferred to work alone; left to its own devices, it could experiment, evaluate, and refine its programs on its own timeframe. Its ideas often departed from conventional wisdom. It has pulled at the realm of experts and tried to bring everything to the people—medicine, agriculture, access to capital, even consciousness. In addition to its strong base of committed staff, it has been aided by a core group of international supporters—academics, donors, politicians and others—who believe in the idea of BRAC as much as BRAC's ideas. This faith and the resources it mobilizes lets BRAC develop as an organization and concentrate on its own agenda, rather than move from one donor's whim to another. These supporters are also the ones who urge BRAC to have a voice in the global dialogue. Few can speak with comparable experience; BRAC has as much of a responsibility as an opportunity to participate in the conversations and influence the development of policies.

BRAC's path to its current size and scope has not been without challenges and setbacks. In moments when donors or global health experts expressed doubt in BRAC's plans, Sir Fazle Hasan Abed, the BRAC team, and its supporters have leveraged BRAC's track record to secure the resources needed to get past the critical "proof of concept" phase. Sometimes it's even had to rely on its own resources, such as when it decided to launch a program in Afghanistan and could not find a donor to fund its initial plans. But in several cases, once it demonstrates that an idea can be done, such as teaching mothers to make oral rehydration for their children with diarrhea, or community health volunteers administering tuberculosis treatment, others are willing to contribute to replicating the success. But BRAC must provide the spark and initial kindling to ignite the effort.

For most working in global health, "going to scale" is the looming challenge. But when a visitor asks one of the many long-time staff member at BRAC to talk about the development of the TB program, he'll tell a story from the early 1980s, about sitting on the ground with a group of *shebikas*, listening to them talk about their experiences visiting households to talk about *jokkha* [colloquial term for TB]. The visitor will listen intently to the recollection, as it is told with the warm smile that a good memory will bring. The story-teller finishes, lost in thought for a moment, and then adds, as an afterthought, "And then we scaled up." As if the process of moving from 264 patients to 100,000 is trivial and does not require its own explanation. And yet, this is the formula for BRAC stories; they contain many, many intricacies at the pilot level, but once they enter the machinery in the scale-up phase, the destination is clear. Scale is second nature for BRAC; it's getting the idea right at the earlier stages that sets everything else in motion.

In 2004, as part of its dialogue with the government of Afghanistan about implementing community-based DOTS, several senior Afghan officials visited Bangladesh to see BRAC's program. After visiting the field, they commented, "It is easy to run a TB program here." After all, Bangladesh has a very dense, relatively homogeneous population living for the most part in flat terrain, with relative security and stability. As BRAC International expands, its leaders wryly comment on the "luxury of working in Bangladesh" as they encounter new challenges abroad, such as the constant mobility of populations (in Uganda and Southern Sudan), government restrictions on NGOs and visa challenges, and finding trained and competent local staff. Donor representatives, government officials, and even communities themselves often regard BRAC teams with the suspicion given to newcomers, unfamiliar with the organization and skeptical that their experience in Bangladesh can translate to the local context. But BRAC has a long history of working in the face of such doubts. "Proof of concept" can apply to more than one kind of skepticism, and producing results is as persuasive today as it was 40 years ago. Often,

BRAC's initial efforts abroad are led by experienced Bangladeshi staff, but as BRAC hires more and more locally and builds the management and leadership capacity for these individuals to run the programs themselves, the programs evolve and cease to be a transported model shipped in from Bangladesh. They acquire their own distinctly local character.

Which leaves BRAC with an existential question: What does it mean to be part of BRAC? What is the BRAC DNA that should permeate throughout its widespread programs, tying all its many activities together? No doubt, part of the answer is the mantra, "Small is beautiful, but large is necessary." Whether a result of having the "luxury" to grow up in a country inherently prone to scale, BRAC's commitment to "health for all" and relentless pursuit of its realization are no doubt central to what BRAC "is" and "will be," despite its growing international presence and identity. The more pressing question is what the sequel will be to the stories that now end with, "And then we scaled up."

BRAC's TB program is just one of the stories, but one that illustrates the layers of complexities and considerations in translating an idea like community-based volunteers overseeing daily treatment into a large-scale program with many partners. While the delivery system itself requires careful management, without the overarching enterprise such as the information systems, the financial office, and the wealth of ongoing development efforts in other sectors, like microfinance, education, and agriculture, the BRAC TB program would have been much more difficult to implement.

Hindsight is never perfect, and sitting in the bustling BRAC office now, finding time to reflect on the 27 years of TB programming is a challenge. Even on paper, we find it easier to describe the activities than to analyze what we did. We hope that our audience draws its own conclusions, and sees from this history the potential for new innovations that will be the inspiration for the next generation of programs that see the realization of "health for all" and "a world free of poverty."

11.1 Digging into "And then we scaled up"

The huge coverage gaps and unmet health needs that exist globally must be addressed. To this end, we will explore a few of the major themes on scale that we think BRAC's experience in TB highlights, and which will be useful to others. In other parts of the book, particularly in Chapters 3 and 4, we discuss necessary components of the pilot and scale-up phase. In addition to the conclusions that we've offered throughout, we would like to highlight a few of the key areas of particular challenge or importance for others engaged in their own efforts to scale up. We would summarize these as follows:

- Scientific evidence is important to justify scale up;
- Staff at all levels must be motivated, supported, and retained;
- Scaling up requires resources of many types and usually, from many sources;
- Effective partnerships facilitate growth, but require transparent and frequent communication;
- Improvement is a continuous process.

In global health, speaking from a solid base of scientific evidence enables a program to dispel doubt and can attract new partnerships or donors. There are many examples of BRAC's use of results to influence others, from its insistence on maintaining the patient bond when signing a memorandum of understanding with the NTP of Bangladesh or in recent years with regards to community-based DOTS in Afghanistan. While BRAC programs embody its values, it has recognized the weakness of trying to compel others on moral grounds. Hard numbers and well conducted studies get far more traction. Investments in evaluation are a longer-term effort; for innovative program designs, the payoff from having the data in hand accrues over time.

It is difficult for any program to produce good results when staff turnover levels are high. This is particularly true for scale up, when a program needs experienced people to expedite the learning process for new staff. Many times the conversation of staff retention focuses on senior leaders and frontline staff, but a shortage of mid-level managers can also cripple a program's efforts to scale. When planning for scale up, program leaders should consider how they will motivate and support staff during the growth period. BRAC uses a number of formal and informal processes to empower staff continuously.

Scaling up is inherently resource intensive, no matter how lean a program may seem. When preparing to scale, programs should consider what pools of resources exist in their ecosystem that could be leveraged to produce better or faster results. BRAC has the benefit of an extensive number of development programs that assisted the TB program scale up in two significant ways: first, they had created a palpable community presence and efficient vehicle for health delivery through the village organization formation and ongoing activity. The TB program is able to tap into these networks instead of having to invest the time to create community relationships on its own. Secondly, other programs offered reserves of staff, particularly at that crucial field and district-level manager, who needed only basic instruction to begin their work. Already familiar with BRAC operations, they could be trusted to manage local activities and required less supervision from the central team.

Many organizations will lack the depth of BRAC's internal resources, but partnerships are another important tool for scale up. BRAC's program relied on the government health system for its clinical services and medical expertise, not to mention medications and laboratory supplies. The public sector infrastructure was already in place before BRAC scaled, providing a national framework for BRAC to link its TB programs with as it grew.

BRAC's experience indicates that partnerships require investments of their own. Honest and frequent communication is not always easy but creates the kind of trust necessary for the coordination and flexibility that scale up requires. Communication at the high levels does not always trickle down; programs must be prepared to approach the individuals working in the public sector facilities and field and build relationships at this level as well. Experienced staff can play a critical role in transmitting the sense of partnership to others.

It's never too late or too soon to improve. Programs should constantly evolve. Change can be inspired on many levels, from the insights of field staff to the wisdom of technical experts. Scaling up is a process of experimentation, and programs should build their plans with the flexibility to enable the healthy refinement that the process can allow. Decentralization is one strategy BRAC uses to empower staff to take initiative in testing new ideas and problem solving, with regular supervision from divisional or central level managers to create a mechanism for institutionalizing promising new practices.

11.2 Reflections on being big

Scaling up a delivery system is difficult, but building an organization capable of managing multiple projects in various stages of pilot, scaling up, and sustaining at scale is even more complex. These observations are meant more as long-term reflections; from the perspective of what actions should be implemented early on to nurture the slow capabilities that may at first seem unnecessary or invisible, but build an organizational foundation strong enough to sustain at scale and weather future challenges.

Organizations can function without systems, but not at scale

Having Sir Fazle Hasan Abed at the helm for the entirety of BRAC's history has been critical. Even today, his thoughtful guidance continues to serve as BRAC's compass. But even a brilliant leader cannot run an organization like BRAC without a sophisticated management structure to support him. Accountability, supervision, performance data, thorough accounting, and even communications strategy or risk management cannot be accomplished by individuals. They require departments and protocols, "bureaucracies" and "administrative obstacles" even. BRAC can scale like a well-oiled machine because it has constructed the machine. It cannot operate without a talented driver, but without the apparatus, the driver cannot move far or fast. Abed benefited from invaluable assistance of operations mastermind Aminul Alam, who helped build many of the develop programs and create their internal structures. Small programs can rely on charismatic leadership and dedicated staff, but those looking to scale should be quite deliberate in codifying processes and building an organizational system even in their early activities.

Capacity building is continuous

Many implementers get stuck in the trenches. Given the overwhelming health needs in developing countries, this is hardly surprising. There is rarely time for learning in these situations. And yet, ultimately, the failure to make time for learning retards an organization's capability and threatens its ability to both retain staff with natural curiosity and to generate innovative ideas and new solutions. Time and opportunities for learning are essential and must be embedded in any organization. This is true not just for senior leadership, or even promising junior staff, but at every level, especially for a health program like BRAC's where only 1% of the team sits in the head office. Decentralized decision-making has great potential, but only when staff have been trained how to respond effectively and in accordance with BRAC's policies and priorities. BRAC ensures regular training for all its employees, in technical areas and management. Leadership is supportive of staff leaving to pursue fellowships and higher education; many write their theses on topics related to BRAC's program and then return to the program with a new set of skills to contribute. They may even go on to work at other institutions in health and development, creating new opportunities for BRAC to build relationships.

Finally, part of capacity building is building a sense of shared mission and organizational ownership. The "BRAC DNA" does not reside primarily in the headquarters; it should be present in the actions of leaders like Sir Fazle Hasan Abed as well as every one of BRAC's 89,000 *shebikas*. Staff members and employees should feel a responsibility to uphold and promote the BRAC brand and model its values in their work. To do this, BRAC must communicate a common vision across its staff that includes them. Cultivating a strong sense of organizational identity, a "we," helps a large organization maintain coherence in its activities. Culture is living and must be nourished and sustained continuously like any other capacity. A common history or set of challenges, no matter how compelling, is not enough at scale.

Partnerships are not easy, but they are essential

Particularly in its early years, BRAC was a bit of a maverick in the development world and preferred to work alone. This can no longer be the case. In TB alone, BRAC has over 44 partners to consider; other programs can list dozens of other organizations with similar activities and priorities to what they are doing. BRAC can continue to think about how to fill the gaps in the existing system, but it must work with other players to best serve the people.

One of the great things about partnerships is that sometimes they allow an organization to focus on what it wants to do. BRAC is very good at community-based health activities; it has less interest in complex clinical services (BRAC Afghanistan being an exception). Many of its TB partners excel in clinical services; BRAC can leverage their expertise to build its own, or link its community-based programs to their clinical services, ensuring patients receive high-quality services through the entire care cycle.

The landscapes everywhere are increasingly crowded. Private sector growth, increasing access to technology and mobility, and epidemiological transitions are ongoing. These challenges require a range of capabilities that are difficult for one organization to acquire and apply simultaneously. Partnerships provide another option that allows BRAC to continue to utilize its specific set of skills in an effective way.

Partnerships do not organically become strong. Organizational entropy tends towards working alone. For a partnership to flourish, it needs sustenance, through meetings, constant and honest communication, mutual respect and accountability, and most critically, trust. These components are particularly important for a public-private partnership. The balance between influencing policy, empowering the government, demanding quality and ensuring effective implementation is can be difficult particularly for an organization of BRAC's size. Working in health with and under nine governments worldwide, BRAC is seeing the difference that government support, trust, and partnership can make in their ease and effectiveness of operations. Despite these challenges of partnerships, they enable new frontiers of expansion and possibility, and therefore are worth the effort.

There is always room to improve

While there is much wisdom in the saying, "Don't let the perfect be the enemy of the good," an organization should always be striving to improve its model. Even in the rare case that perfection is somehow hypothetically attained, the pace of change in today's world means that within moments, the fit will be at least slightly obsolete. Programs should assume that models will evolve and build the space and encouragement for that growth into their processes. Good data systems are an important source of information about how well a program is working, as is formal research and external evaluation. None of these replace the need for field visits and conversations with frontline staff and, of course, the people themselves.

Do, but also inspire and teach

Implementing is in many ways the most basic element of scale. But in terms of long-term impact, convincing and enabling others to adapt effective models, and institutionalize them in policy, potentially has a much greater impact. What is clear from the decades of development programs is that just building something good is not enough to ensure its replication or dissemination. In Afghanistan, BRAC persuaded the National Tuberculosis Program to let it implement community-based DOTS in its own working areas, and within a few years, the Ministry of Health added community-based DOTS as a required activity in the nation's basic package of health services. BRAC could disappear tomorrow, and patients would continue to have that service available. Similar opportunities exist at the organizational, national, and global level; but these will require BRAC to craft a new strategy, one that's more encompassing in its goals, less intent on doing things itself, and more confident in enabling others to act, not just going at it alone. The TB model in particular has great applicability to other contexts and conditions. BRAC has shown that scale is achievable, not just in the "luxury" of Bangladesh, but increasingly in a diverse number of contexts worldwide. Scale's complexity is manageable, and small failures, when one learns from them, better equip an organization to meet whatever is waiting around the corner. Faith in scalability, and moreover, the responsibility to scale up because of the magnitude of need confronting us, must catalyze action.

Appendixes

Appendix A

Brief History of Modern TB Control

BRAC's tuberculosis (TB) program is best understood if put into the context of TB control in the modern era. Several publications have summarized the major milestones of the 20th century (Lonnroth et al., 2009; Raviglione and Pio, 2002; Arnadottir, 2009). The 1940s and World War II mark the beginning of a much more global perspective on public health. During this period, public health programs began to focus on controlling or eradicating a single communicable disease (a strategy termed "vertical"). Priority was increasingly placed on addressing those conditions with a known effective treatment or vaccination or on vectors for which there were insecticides or other control measures. Some countries began anti-TB mass vaccination campaigns with bacillus Calmette-Guerin (BCG), though its value in reducing incidence was later disputed (TB Reider, 2010). Streptomycin, a drug that continues to serve as a first-line treatment for TB even today, was discovered in 1944, catalyzing TB control efforts globally as it became widely available in the following years (Raviglione and Pio, 2002). In 1947, the World Health Organization (WHO) recognized TB as a global priority, based on its prevalence and contribution to the burden of disease (Raviglione and Pio, 2002). New medications, isoniazid and pyrazinamide, were discovered in 1952 and 1954 respectively, creating a more powerful combination therapy (Institute of Medicine, 2009). Armed with improving treatments, in the 1950s, the approach to TB control became increasingly medicalized. "Single purpose machinery," such as TB clinics (where patients could come without infecting others) and mass screenings were implemented, largely by wealthy countries who had resources to devote to the efforts (Raviglione and Pio, 2002). Standard treatment regimens lasted 12-24 months with complete bed rest, often in a hospital or sanatorium (Arnadottir, 2009, 79, 167). Relapse was very common and patients were recommended for screening every 3-6 months for several years (or even life) (Arnadottir, 2009, 79). Drug susceptibility testing was considered critical, therefore limiting treatment only to those whose facilities were capable of providing these services. In the 1960s, researchers in India found that the rates of active TB in the family members of patients receiving ambulatory care did not differ significantly that those of patients who were hospitalized, creating exciting potential for expanding ambulatory care options (Kamat et al., 1966).

The tuberculosis services that had been developed in wealthy countries could not be implemented in most poor developing countries. Mass screening programs were seen as prohibitively expensive and, more crucially, the medications to treat TB were costly (Raviglione and Pio, 2002). Wealthy countries benefited from the general improvements that they experienced during the 1950s as well; studies on the decline of TB control in advanced economies largely conclude that TB was declining even prior to the introduction of these control efforts. Significant economic improvement and social reform resulted in improved living conditions, nutritional status, and poverty reduction, all of which combined to further reduce the spread of TB (Lonnroth et al, 2009).

In the 1960s, with the declining rates of TB in many countries, there was a global shift in strategy towards integrating TB services into general health services (Raviglione and Pio, 2002). As combination therapy became more widely practiced and studied, treatment recommendations changed greatly and patient outcomes improved. Typical regimens included high doses of combination therapy during the "intensive phase" to significantly reduce the bacilli load and the "continuation phase" to ensure that persistent bacilli are eliminated, and the patient was completely cured. New drugs reduced the relapse rate, eliminated the need for drug susceptibility testing as a standard part of treatment, and shortened the treatment course (Arnadottir, 2009, 80-86). Rifampicin, discovered in 1963, also enhanced the efficacy of treatment when taken in combination with the other medications (Institute of Medicine, 2009). During this time diagnosis was simplified as researchers found that sputum microscopy reliably identified most infectious cases of TB, reducing reliance on the more expensive and less available method utilizing radiology (Arnadottir, 2009, 113).

Many studies were reporting resistance to medications, linked with monotherapy or missed dosages of treatment. Ensuring that patients adhered to the treatment regimen, particularly during the "intensive" phase (the first two months during which rifampicin was administered), became a new research priority. In settings using daily injections of streptomycin, patients were already attending the clinic every day; asking them to take their oral medications during the visit so that it could be directly observed was a minor change some believed would enhance adherence and prevent the emergence of drug resistance significantly (Ray and Wilkinson, 1995). Increasingly supervision of treatment became a recommended practice for the intensive phase of treatment.

Much of this research was conducted in developing countries. However, these pilot programs were islands in settings that still largely lacked the capacity and resources to implement robust TB control programs. The global trends of the 1950s had continued: high- and middle-income countries observed continuing decreases in TB prevalence, while in low-income countries prevalence remained high with slower rates of reduction. Global interest in tuberculosis control waned in the 1970s and 1980s, as TB became increasingly a concern only of poor countries (Raviglione and Pio, 2002). Halfdan Mahler, former Director General of the WHO, believed that public health initiatives such as those for TB could not be implemented without a proper health services infrastructure. Under his leadership, in 1978 the WHO co-sponsored the Declaration of Alma Ata that emphasized the importance of primary health care to focus attention on the basic health needs. Consequently, many TB programs were dissolved into larger initiatives of health sector reforms.

Much would change in the 1980s that would motivate the world to renew its commitment to TB control. Many experts believed that a six month "short-course" treatment (which included rifampicin) was not feasible in developing countries settings and to prevent resistance and were against promoting or facilitating its availability. However, a promising pilot study conducted in Tanzania 1979-1981 demonstrated that a nine-month therapy with rifampicin produced clinical outcomes comparable to the standard 12-18 month treatment that lacked rifampicin. Cure rates of over 80% were achieve when adequate drug supply was ensured and there was full supervision of drugs during the intensive phase (Raviglione and Pio, 2002). All treatment was provided on an outpatient basis, a promising practice given the limited availability of health facilities in many developing countries.

When these results were further demonstrated in Malawi, Mozambique, Benin and Nicaraguain the TB collaborative programs of International Union against Tuberculosis and Lung Disease (the Union), the evidence that TB could be effectively treated with short-course therapy on an outpatient basis in resource-constrained settings was compelling (Enarson 1991). These findings would eventually become the basis for the global guidelines, which in 1982 recommended a six-month treatment course. However, rifampicin and pyrazinamide were still relatively expensive compared to older TB drugs, and many countries opted to continue using older and longer regimens, despite the benefits of the short-course regimen. The calculus changed as HIV emerged. First described in 1981, HIV's effects on the immune system put people living with HIV at an elevated risk for TB, an "opportunistic infection." It is the leading cause of morbidity and mortality for people living with HIV (WHO website, 2011). In those countries where there was a significant prevalence of HIV, incidence of TB also rose in the general population. With no active investments for many years, the world was ill equipped for this surge in new cases. Even wealthy countries, such as the United States, found that their crumbling programs lacked the capacity to control the rising incidence rates (Raviglione and Pio, 2002).

Creating guidance for HIV and TB control that was feasible given resource constraints became a priority for a few institutions, including the Union, who in 1986 published the first edition of "the orange guide," with guidelines for treatment control and treatment. They recommended that in developing countries, patients be hospitalized for the first two months (of the 12 month treatment), given their difficulty in accessing facilities for daily observed therapy (Arnadottir, 2009, 236). In urban areas or for patients with access to reliable transportation, care was recommended on an outpatient basis.

In 1990, informed by the results of the collaborative TB programs of the Union, the World Bank released a report declaring short-course therapy for TB one of the most cost-effective interventions available, comparable to vaccination campaigns and oral rehydration solution (Arnadottir, 2009, 146). The higher cure rates achieved by the six-month regimen with rifampicin and pyrazinamide resulted in a lower cost per patient cured than the longer regimens (US \$314 compared to US \$368) (CDC, 1990). Reports from programs in developing countries sharing successful program experiences, including BRAC, further proved that TB control could be implemented effectively in any setting, with the proper resources and strategies (Chowdhury et al, 1991).

At this point, however, TB control globally was largely in a state of disrepair, under-funded and with limited activity. A WHO assessment found only 10 countries in the world with a functional TB control program and only US \$16 million of external financing was going to TB control in developing countries (Raviglione and Pio, 2002). In response to these findings, the World Health Assembly set ambitious targets in an effort to motivate countries to bolster these programs and tackle TB in earnest. In 1991, they announced global targets of identifying 75% of cases and achieving an 85% cure rate by 2000. In 1995 the WHO declared the strategy developed in the Union's collaborative programs as the "DOTS" strategy, for Directly Observed Therapy, Short-course. These five components of this strategy were: political commitment with increased and sustained financing; case detection through quality assured bacteriology; standardized treatment with supervision and patient support; an effective drug supply and management system; and monitoring and evaluation systems and impact measurement.

Widespread adoption and implementation of the DOTS strategy created a need to recognize new sources of treatment supervisors (Arnadottir, 2009,

241). The traditional facility-based model taxed limited human resources and created barriers for poor patients. Indeed, a multi-country study in 1992 found that the two strongest predictors of adherence were family income and type of dwelling (Arnadottir, 2009, 223). Respected community leaders and family members became common DOTS providers, enabling patients to visit the facility less frequently while preserving the mechanism for adherence (Arnadottir, 2009, 241).

In 2001, the WHO created the Global DOTS Expansion Plan to support TB control scale-up in the 22 "high burden countries," including Bangladesh, which accounted for (and continue to account for) 80% of the global burden of TB. Discovering that these countries lacked the resources to finance programming internally, the WHO advocated for an additional US $1-2 billion per year for TB control. In 2000, external financing for TB in developing countries had grown to just US $190 million (Raviglione and Pio, 2002).

The Global Fund to Fight AIDS, TB, and Malaria (Global Fund) created a pool of public and private financing, changing the dialog around global health overnight. From 2002-2010, US $21.7 billion was granted to 150 governments for disease control and treatment (Global Fund, 2011). About one fifth (US $4.3 billion) was dedicated to TB control programming. These resources were accompanied by additional bilateral and private financing. For example, in 2006, US $1.9 billion in funding was directed to TB programming in the 22 high burden countries (Marais et al, 2010). By 2008, virtually all countries had adopted the DOTS strategy. Case detection was over 60% and treatment success around 87%. Experts estimated that from 1995-2008, DOTS led to the cure of 36 million people and averted 6 million deaths (Marais et al, 2010). Tuberculosis, however, remains a major cause of death in low and middle income countries; in 2009, there were 9.4 million cases of TB and 1.8 million deaths (Kranzer, 2011; Lonnroth et al, 2010).

Tubercle bacilli can become resistant to drugs that are effective in its treatment, and can be caused by interruptions in treatment (i.e. missing weeks of medication). Adherence to and completion of the treatment course is the best way to prevent resistance. Multidrug resistant (MDR) TB refers to strains that are resistant to first-line drugs (isoniazid and rifampicin) and require other medications that are much more expensive (US $20 for first-line course of treatment compared to US $3,500 for second-line treatment) and often have more severe side effects (Bartlett, 2006). The drug costs for the first-line course of treatment is US $20, whereas the drug cost for second-line treatment is US $3,500, or 175 times more. Current treatment guidelines recommend a mainly ambulatory course of treatment of at least 20 months, and in practice management of MDR TB often involves hospitalization, particularly during the intensive phase (WHO, 2010). Experts estimate that there are 440,000 new cases of MDR TB annually. Close to 250,000 occurred in the 27 countries considers as "high burden," with just 16% appropriately notified as MDR TB (WHO, 2011).[1] In 1998, the DOTS strategy was revised into "DOTS-plus." The updated strategy acknowledged the importance of empowering patients and communities as part of TB control activities. Reducing stigma, increasing awareness, generating social support, and implementing creative incentive schemes such as BRAC's may help patients better seek services and adhere to treatment and thereby reduce the incidence of TB.

Though there have been efforts to significantly reduce the costs of second-line, most poor countries, still cannot afford the needed quantity of these medications. There are many activities to build the capabilities to diagnose drug resistance. Recently, strains of extremely drug resistant (XDR) TB (strains that have resistance to these second-line drugs plus fluoroquinolone and at least one type of injectable drug) have been identified, especially in southern Africa, the epicenter of the global AIDS epidemic and home to high levels of TB-HIV co-infection. XDR TB is often fatal or requires treatment that is not available in resource-limited settings. Treatment of XDR TB, even if clinically achievable, will be beyond the reach of most countries.

In 2010, US $2.6 billion was available for TB treatment, a marked increase from a decade before, but still far below the WHO's estimates for what would be needed to meet the current targets of halving global burden from its 1990 rate by 2015 (i.e. a global prevalence of under 150 per 100,000 and fewer than 15 deaths per 100,000 cases per year) (Marais et al, 2010). In addition to funding for service delivery, investments in research and development are needed to improve diagnostic tools and more effective drugs and vaccines. Promising breakthroughs have been made for rapid diagnosis of MDR TB using line probe assays and other new methods. Many of the emerging technologies will require adaptations and price reductions before they are feasible for developing countries to adopt. It is clear from the recent history of TB control that building programs with strong mechanisms for adherence to prevent drug resistance, both for individual patients and population health (as others can acquire drug resistant strains through contact with infectious patients), is key. While building capacity to diagnose and treat these conditions is critical, preventing drug resistance through

---

[1] WHO recommends that all patients have drug sensitivity testing conducted at the start of treatment, but recognizes that this is currently infeasible in high burden countries (WHO, 2010). In Bangladesh, for example, new sputum smear-positive cases only undergo drug sensitivity testing if they fail the six-month treatment (remain sputum smear-positive; ideally at the conclusion of the two-month intensive phase, patients would test sputum smear-negative). Previously treated patients receive drug sensitivity testing if they are sputum smear-positive at five months. See Chapter 5 for more details.

strong basic TB programs promoting high levels of case detection and adherence should remain a primary strategy (WHO, 2011). Many low-income countries even question the value of these new diagnostics to patients, if drugs are unaffordable.

Current discussions on TB control largely focus on medical interventions. However, the experience of advanced economies during the last century points to the importance of social, economic, and demographic factors in reducing the burden of TB (Lonnroth et al, 2009). The growing trend of urbanization creates dense living conditions and overcrowding where TB can flourish. Malnutrition and poverty create vulnerability to the disease. Trends in behaviors and environmental factors, such as smoking and indoor air pollution, influence the incidence of TB (Lonnroth et al., 2009). Some experts estimate that 50% of the TB incidence in India is related to smoking, and diabetes accounts for 20% of cases (Lawn and Zumla, 2011). Migration, domestic and international, allows TB to travel. True control of TB likely will require attention to these broader factors as well to reduce incidence.

For more information on the history of TB control and the global context, we recommend these recent, open-access publications as starting points:

- *The Lancet* series on tuberculosis, 2010.
  http://www.thelancet.com/series/tuberculosis

- Arnadottir, T. 2009. Tuberculosis and Public Health. Policies and Principles in Tuberculosis Control. Paris, France: International Union Against TB and Lung Disease.[2]

- Stop TB Partnership: http://www.stoptb.org/global/plan/

- Raviglione, M.C., Pio, A. 2002. Evolution of WHO policies for tuberculosis control, 1948-2001. *The Lancet*. 359; 775-780.

- Lawn, S.D., Zumla, A. 2011. Tuberculosis. *The Lancet*. 378; 57-72.

---

[2] For article URL, please see listing in references.

Appendix B

About BRAC

In 1972, BRAC began its work in Bangladesh by providing relief after a war for independence. Its vision is a world free from all forms of exploitation and discrimination where everyone has the opportunity to realize their potential. Over the years, the organization has evolved and grown, guided by the principles of innovation, integrity, inclusiveness, and effectiveness.

BRAC is a development organization dedicated to the alleviation of poverty by empowering the poor to bring about positive change in their own lives. BRAC's approach encompasses services in areas of education, health care, social and economic empowerment, finance and enterprise development, human rights and legal aid, agriculture and food security, as well as environmental sustainability and disaster preparedness.

BRAC organizes the poor, especially women, and provide platforms for them to come together, access services, exchange information, analyze and raise awareness on economic, social, legal, gender and other issues concerning their daily lives and their communities. Its social enterprises integrated with the various development programs form crucial linkages that increase the productivity of its members' assets and labor and generate surplus for the organization, allowing both those BRAC supports and BRAC to be increasingly self-reliant.

In 2002, BRAC began to expand internationally. While it continues to rely on its integrated approach, it is rapidly exploring new strategies to tackle the distinct challenges of poverty its finds on the ground. Worldwide, BRAC touches the lives of more than 138 million people.

References

Afghanistan Country Coordinating Mechanism. 2007. Consolidating TB control activities in line with the new Stop TB Strategy. Received by the Global Fund to fight AIDS, TB, and malaria. AFG-809-G07-T. http://portfolio.theglobalfund.org/en/Grant/List/AFG. Accessed on July 6, 2011.

Afghanistan Country Coordinating Mechanism. 2009. Proposal for Round 10 of the GFATM. Received by the Global Fund to fight AIDS, TB, and Malaria. http://portfolio.theglobalfund.org/en/Country/Index/AFG. Accessed on July 6, 2011.

Afsana, K. 2010. Scaling up BRAC's maternal, neonatal and child health interventions in Bangladesh. In *From one to many. Scaling up health programs in low income countries*, edited by Cash, R.A., Chowdhury, A.M.R., Smith, G.B., and Ahmed, F., 59-74. Dhaka: The University Press Limited.

Afsana, K., Ahmed, S.M., Mayeed, M., Roy, R.D., Karim, F. 1998. Women, workload, and the women's health and development programme: are women overburdened? *Research Monograph series* (11). BRAC Research and Evaluation Division: Dhaka, Bangladesh. http://www.bracresearch.org/monographs/mono_11.pdf. Accessed on July 1, 2011.

Ahmad, K. 2004. Health and money in Afghanistan. *The Lancet*. 364; 1301-02. http://www.thelancet.com/journals/lancet/article/PIIS0140-6736(04)17208-5/fulltext.

Ahmed, S.M. 2008. Taking health care where the community is: the story of the shasthya shebikas of BRAC in Bangladesh. *BRAC University Journal*. 5; 39-45.

Ahmed, S.M. 2010. Revisiting the Shasthya Shebika model of BRAC's EHC: Fit for Community Health Care in the 21st Century? BRAC internal document.

Akhter, Z. 2010. "Understanding shasthya kormi, a vital ingredient of BRAC's Health Program." Master's thesis, James P. Grant School of Public Health, BRAC University.

Amin, R., Chowdhury, S.A., Kamal, G.M., Chowdhury, J. 1989. Community health services and health care utilization in rural Bangladesh. *Social Science and Medicine*. 29:1343-1349.

Angeles, G., Lance, P., Barden-O'Fallon, J., Islam, N., Mahbub, A.Q.M., Nazem, N.I. 2009. The 2005 Census and mapping of slums in Bangladesh: design, select results, and application. *The International Journal of Health Geographics*.

Arnadottir, T. 2009. Tuberculosis and Public Health. Policies and Principles in Tuberculosis Control. Paris, France: International Union Against TB and Lung Disease. http://www.tbrieder.org/publications/books_english/rm22038.pdf. Accessed on June 28, 2011.

Atun, R., Bataringaya, J. 2011. Building a durable response to HIV/AIDS: implications for health systems. *Journal of Acquired Immune Deficiency Syndrome*. 57; S91-S95.

Bangladesh Country Coordinating Mechanism. 2003. Bangladesh TB Proposal to GFATM. Received by the Global Fund to Fight AIDS, TB, and Malaria. BAN-304-G02-T. URL. http://portfolio.theglobalfund.org/en/Grant/List/BAN. Accessed on July 1, 2011.

Bangladesh Country Coordinating Mechanism. 2005. Bangladesh TB Proposal for 5th round of GFATM. Received by the Global Fund to Fight AIDS, TB, and Malaria. BAN-506-G04-T. URL. http://portfolio.theglobalfund.org/en/Grant/List/BAN. Accessed on July 1, 2011.

Bangladesh Country Coordinating Mechanism. 2005. Bangladesh TB Proposal for 5th round of GFATM. Received by the Global Fund to Fight AIDS, TB, and Malaria. BAN-506-G04-T. URL. http://portfolio.theglobalfund.org/en/Grant/List/BAN. Accessed on July 1, 2011.

Bangladesh Country Coordinating Mechanism. 2007. CCM Bangladesh Round 8 Tuberculosis Proposal with Health Systems Strengthening Cross-cutting Interventions. Received by the Global Fund to Fight AIDS, TB, and Malaria. BAN-809-G10-T. URL. http://portfolio.theglobalfund.org/en/Grant/List/BAN. Accessed on July 1, 2011.

Bangladesh Country Coordinating Mechanism. 2010. Round 10 Proposal to GFATM. Received by the Global Fund to Fight AIDS, TB, and Malaria. URL: http://portfolio.theglobalfund.org/en/Country/Index/BAN. Accessed on July 1, 2011.

Bangladesh National Tuberculosis Program. 2006. 2005 Annual Report. Dhaka: BRAC Health Program.

Bangladesh National Tuberculosis Program. 2010. Annual Report 2010. Dhaka: BRAC Health Program.

Bangladesh National Tuberculosis Program. 2011. NTP Factsheet on 2010 MIS data.

Bangsberg, D.R., Deeks, S.G. 2010. Spending more to save more: interventions to promote adherence. *Annals of internal medicine*. 152; 54-56.

Bartlett, J. 2006. The Potential Disaster of Extensively Drug Resistant TB. *Clinicians' Biosecurity Network*. Nov 10. http://www.upmc-cbn.org/offline/2006/11_November_2006/cbnreport_111006.html. Accessed on 26 June, 2011.

Behforouz, H., Farmer, P.E., Mukherjee, J. 2004. From Directly Observed Therapy to Accompangeteurs: Enhancing AIDS treatment outcomes in Haiti and in Boston. *Clinical Infectious Disease*. 38; S429-436.

Berman, P.A., Gwatkin, D.R., Burger, S.E. 1985. Community-based health workers: head start or false start towards health for all? *Social Science and Medicine*. 25; 443-459.

Berwick, D. Improvement tip: want a new level of performance? Get a new system. Institute of Healthcare Improvement. http://www.ihi.org/IHI/Topics/

Improvement/ImprovementMethods/ImprovementStories/ImprovementTip WantaNewLevelofPerformanceGetaNewSystem.htm. Accessed on July 6, 2011.

Bohmer, R.M.J. 2005. Medicine's service challenge: blending custom and standard care. *Health Care Management Review.* 30; 322-330.

Bohmer, R.M.J. 2010. Fixing health care on the front lines. *Harvard Business Review.* April, 62-69.

Bornstein, D., Susan, D. 2010. Social entrepreneurship: what everyone needs to know. New York: Oxford University Press.

BRAC. 2010. BRAC Annual Report 2009. www.brac.net/oldsite/useruploads/files/brac-ar-2009.pdf. Accessed on July 1, 2011.

BRAC. 2011. BRAC Annual Report 2010. http://issuu.com/brac/docs/brac-annual-report-2010. Accessed on July 13, 2011.

Brinkof Martin, W.G., Dabis, F., Myer, L., Bangsberg, D.R., Boulle, A., Nash, D., Schechter, M., Laurent, C., Keiser, O., May, M., Sprinz, E., Egger, M., Anglaret, X. 2008. Early loss of HIV-infected patients on potent antiretroviral therapy programmes in lower-income countries. *Bulletin of the World Health Organization.* 86; 559-567.

Buse, K., Hamer, A.M. 2007. Seven habits of highly effective global public-private health partnerships: practice and potential. *Social Science and Medicine.* 64: 259-271.

Chesney, M. 2006. The elusive gold standard: future perspectives for HIV adherence assessment and intervention. *Journal of AIDS.* 43; S149-155.

Chowdhury, A.M.R., Alam, A., Chowdhury, S.A., Ahmed, J. 1992. Tuberculosis Control in Bangladesh. *The Lancet.* 339; 1181-1182.

Chowdhury, A.M.R., Alam, M.A., Ahmed, J. 2006. Development knowledge and experience—from Bangladesh to Afghanistan and beyond. *Bulletin of the World Health Organization* 84; 677-81.

Chowdhury, A.M.R., Chowdhury, S., Islam, M.N., Islam, A., Vaughan, J.P. 1997. Control of tuberculosis by community health workers in Bangladesh. *The Lancet.* 350; 169-172.

Chowdhury, A.M.R., Ishikawa, N., Alam, A., Islam, M.S., Hossain, S., Cash, R.A., Abed, F.H. 1991. Controlling a forgotten disease. Using voluntary health workers for tuberculosis control in rural Bangladesh. *Newsletter of the International Union against TB and Lung Disease.* December: 2-5.

Chowdhury, A.M.R., Vaughan, J.P., Chowdhury, S., Abed, F.H. 1999. Demystifying the control of tuberculosis in rural Bangladesh. In *Tuberculosis—an Interdisciplinary Perspective.* Edited by John M Grange and John Porter. London, Imperial College Press, 379-396.

Donnell, D., Baeten, J.M., Kiarie, J., Thomas, K., Stevens, W., Cohen, C.R., McIntyre, J., Lingappa, J.R., Celum, C. 2010. Heterosexual HIV-1 transmission after initiation of antiretroviral therapy: a prospective cohort analysis. *The Lancet.* June 12; 375(9731): 2092-2098.

Elridge, C., Palmer, N. 2009. Performance-based payment: some reflections on the discourse, evidence and unanswered questions. *Health Policy and Planning*. 24: 160-166.

Enarson, D. 1991. Principles of IUATLD Collaborative Tuberculosis Programmes. *Bulletin of the International Journal against Tuberculosis and Lung Disease*. 66; 195-200.

Faiz, M.D., Hussain, D., Seddiq, M.K., Zhuben, M., Khuram, M.D., Zarabi, A., Andar, A.H. 2011. Knowledge attitude practice (KAP) survey on Tuberculosis (TB) in Afghanistan. Kabul: Ministry of Public Health, General Directorate of Preventive Medicine, Communicable Disease Control Directorate, National TB Program.

Gapminder.org; "The Bangladesh Miracle." http://www. gapminder.org/videos/gapcasts/gapcast-5-bangladesh-miracle. Accessed on July 1, 2011.

Global Fund to fight AIDS, TB, and Malaria. 2011. Portfolio and Grant Performance. http://www.theglobalfund.org/en/performance/grantportfolio/accessed on July 6, 2011.

Global Fund to fight AIDS, TB, and malaria. Technical Review Panel for Round 10. TB control in Bangladesh. 2011. Unpublished report and responses from BCCM.

Hermann, K., van Damme, W., Pariyo, G.W., Schouten, E., Assefa, Y., Cirera, A., Massavon, W. 2009. Community health workers for ART in sub-Sahara Africa: learning from experience—capitalizing on new opportunities. *Human Resources for Health*. 7; 31.

Institute of Medicine. 2009. Addressing the Threat of Drug-Resistant Tuberculosis: A Realistic Assessment of the Challenge: Workshop Summary. Washington, DC: National Academies Press (US); 2009. http://www.ncbi.nlm.nih.gov/books/NBK45001/Bookshelf ID: NBK45001.

International Center for Diarrheal Disease, Bangladesh. 2010. Nationwide tuberculosis prevalence survey in Bangladesh. ICDDRB Health and Science Bulletin Vol. 8, No. 4; 13-17. Principal Investigator: Zaman, K.

Ishikawa, N. Unpublished interviews with shasthya shebikas. Translated by Rifat Mahfuza.

Ishikawa, N. 1992. Use of health volunteers and a group approach for raising health awareness in rural Bangladesh. *Behavioral Medicine*. Special Edition. 281-288.

Islam, A., Wakai, S., Ishikawa, N., Chowdhury, A.M.R., Vaughan, J.P. 2002. Cost effectiveness of community health workers in Bangladesh. *Bulletin of the World Health Organization*. 80; 445-450.

Islam, M.A. 1999. Impact of involving community health workers in tuberculosis control in rural Bangladesh. PhD dissertation, University of Tokyo.

Islam, M.A., Makamura, Y., Wongkhomthong, S., Chowdhury, S.A., Ishikawa, N. 1999. Involvement of community health workers in tuberculosis control in Bangladesh. *Japan Journal of Tropical Medicine and Hygiene*. 27; 167-173.

Islam, N., Chowdhury, A.M.R., Sarker, M. 1991. An evaluation of shasthya shebika. BRAC. Unpublished research report.

Kamat, S.R., Dawson, J.J.Y., Devadatta, S., Fox, W., Janardhanam, B., Radhakrishna, S., Somasundaram, P.R., Stott, H., Velu, S. 1966. A controlled study on the influence of segregation of tuberculosis patients for one year on the attack rate of tuberculosis in a five-year period in close family contacts in South India. *Bulletin of the World Health Organization*. 34; 517-532.

Karim, F., Ahmed, J., Islam, Q.S. 2011. Occupational pulmonary tuberculosis among BRAC community health workers of Trishal, Bangladesh. BRAC Research and Evaluation Division. Manuscript.

Karim, F., Johansson, E., Diwan, V.K., Kulane, A. 2009. Community perceptions of tuberculosis: a qualitative exploration from a gender perspective. *Public Health*. 125; 84-89.

Khan, A.M., Ahmed, S.M. 2011. Current state of the Model Shasthya Shebika of BRAC: a quick exploration of the 'Pilot project for SS Sustainability'. BRAC Research and Evaluation Division.

Khan, M.H., Islam, A.B.M.T., 2010. Expansion of DOTS in urban and public-private mix areas of Bangladesh. *Research and Reports in Tropical Medicine*. 2010; 77-82.

Khan, S.H., Chowdhury, A.M.R., Karim, F., Barua, M.K. 1998. Training and retraining shasthyo shebika: reasons for turnover of community health workers in Bangladesh. *Health Care Supervisor* 17(1): 37-47.

Klugman, J. 2010. The real wealth of nations: pathways to human development. Human Development Report 2010. United Nations Development Programme: New York, USA. http://hdr.undp.org/en/reports/global/hdr2010/chapters/en/. Accessed on July 1, 2011.

Korten, D.C. 1980. Community organization and rural development: a learning process approach. *Public Administration Review*. September/October, 480-511.

Kranzer, K. 2011. Improving TB diagnostics and treatment. *The Lancet*. 377; 1467-1468.

Lonnroth, K., Castro, K., Chakaya, J.M., Chauhan, L.S., Floyd, K., Glaziou, P., Raviglione, M.C. 2010. TB control and elimination 2010-2050: cure, care, and social development. *The Lancet*. 375, 1814-1829.

Lonnroth, K., Jaramillo, E., Williams, B.G., Dye, C., Raviglione, M. 2009. Drivers of tuberculosis epidemics: the role of risk factors and social determinants. *Social Science & Medicine*. 68; 2240-2246.

Losina, E., Toure, H., Uhler, L.M., Anglaret, X., Paltiel, A.D., Balestre, E., Walensky, R.P., Messou, E., Weinstein, M.C., Dabis, F., Freedberg, K.A. 2009. Cost-effectiveness of preventing lost to follow-up in HIV treatment programs: A Cote d'Ivoire appraisal. *PLOS Medicine*. 6(10); e1000173.

Lovell, C.H. 1992. *Breaking the Cycle of Poverty. The BRAC Strategy*. Dhaka: The University Press Limited.

Low-Beer, D., Afkhami, H., Komatsu, R., Banati, P., Sempala, M., Katz, I., Cutler, J., Schumacher, P., Tran-Ba-Hury, R., Schwartlander, B. 2007. Making Performance-based Funding work for health. *PLOS Medicine*. 4: 1308-1311.

Maher, D., Floyd, K., Sharm, B.V., Jaramillo, E., Nkhoma, W., Nyarko, E., Wilkinson, D. 2003. Community contribution to TB care: practice and policy. Geneva: Stop TB Department, World Health Organization.

Management Sciences for Health. 2005. Stories: A formula for success in Afghanistan: USAID grants and REACH technical assistance. News Room. http://www. msh.org/Afghanistan/news_room/stories/BRAC_NGO_Afghanistan_oct2005. html. Accessed on July 1, 2011.

Marais, B.J., Raviglione, M., Donald, P.R., Harries, A.D., Kritski, A.L., Graham, S.M., El-Saadr, W.M., Harrington, M., Churchyard, G., Mwaba, P., Sanne, I., Kaufmann, S.H.E., Whitty, C.J.M., Atun, R., Zumla, A. 2010. Scale-up of services and research priorities for diagnosis, management, and control of tuberculosis: a call to action. *The Lancet*. 375; 2179-91.

Medecins, Sans Frontieres. 2011. Getting ahead of the wave: lessons for the next decade of the AIDS response. *Access to essential medicines campaign*. http://www. msf.org/ shadomx/apps/fms/fmsdownload.cfm?file_uuid=0ADAF3D0-F526-45F2-B0D5-64E6F37B4F59&siteName=msf. Accessed on July 4, 2011.

Ministry of Public Health, Islamic Republic of Afghanistan. 2005. "A basic package of health services for Afghanistan". Kabul: Ministry of Public Health. http://www. msh.org/afghanistan/pdf/Afghanistan_BPHS_2005_1384.pdf. Accessed on July 11, 2011.

Murray, C.J., Styblo, K., Rouillon, A. 1990. Tuberculosis in developing countries. *Morbidity and Mortality Report Weekly* 39; 561,567-569. http://www.cdc.gov/ mmwr/preview/mmwrhtml/00001729.htm. Accessed on July 1, 2011.

National Institute of Population Research and Training, MEASURE Evaluation, International Center for Diarrheal Disease Research, Bangladesh. 2010. Bangladesh maternal mortality and health care survey. Preliminary results.

National Tuberculosis Control Program, Ministry of Public Health, Afghanistan. 2011. *Annual Report 2010*.

National Tuberculosis Program Afghanistan. 2010. *Annual Report 2009*. http://www. stoptbafghanistan.org/wp-content/uploads/2011/04/Annual-Report-2009.pdf. Accessed on July 6, 2011.

Obermeyer, C.M., Baijal, P., Pegurri, E. 2011. Facilitating HIV disclosure across diverse settings: a review. *American Journal of Public Health*. 101; 1011-23.

Osaki, K. 1995. "Deposit money system in community-based tuberculosis programme in rural Bangladesh." In *Improvement in TB Control in Developing Countries* (II). Edited by Nobukatsu Ishikawa, 67-78. Tokyo: Research Institute of Tuberculosis.

Porter, M.E . 1996. What is strategy? *Harvard Business Review*. Nov-Dec. 61-78.

Porter, M.E., Teisberg Elizabeth Olmsted. 2006. *Redefining health care: creating value-based competition on results*. Boston: Harvard Business School Press.

Public Health Watch. 2006. TB policy in Bangladesh. A civil society perspective. New York: Open Society Institute.

Rahman, M., Tasneem, S. 2008. Determinants of income of the shasthya shebikas: evidence from a pilot MNCH initiative in the Nilpharamari district of Bangladesh. *RED Working Paper*. Number 6.

Rahman, M.M. 2011. "Urban TB Control." Presentation at Urban DOTS Workshop, Dhaka. February 2.

Raviglione, M.C., Pio, A. 2002. Evolution of WHO policies for tuberculosis control, 1948-2001. *The Lancet.* 359; 775-780.

Reichenbach, L., Shimul, S.N. In press. Sustaining health: the role of BRAC's community health volunteers in Bangladesh, Afghanistan, and Uganda. *Research Monograph Series.* Dhaka: BRAC.

Rifat, M., Rusen, I.D., Mahmud, M.H., Nayer, I., Islam, A., Ahmed, F. 2008. From Mosques to classrooms: mobilizing the community to enhance case detection of tuberculosis. *American Journal of Public Health.* 98; 1550-1552.

Rohde, J.E. 2005. *Learning to reach health for all.* Dhaka: The University Press Limited.

Rohde, J.E. and Buiya, A. 2010. Where to from here? Reflections on shasthya shebikas in BRAC. BRAC internal document.

Rosen, S., Fox, M.P., Gill, C.J. 2007. Patient retention in antiretroviral therapy programs in sub-Saharan Africa. A systematic review. *Public Library of Sciences.* 4; 1691-1701.

Salim, M.A.H., Uplekar, M., Daru, P., Aung, M., Declercq, E., Lonnroth, K. 2006. Turning liabilities into resources: informal doctors and tuberculosis control in Bangladesh. *Bulletin of the WHO.* 84; 425-504.

Second Urban Primary Health Care Project. 2010. Introduction. http://www.uphcp.org/index.php/welcome/aboutuphcp. Accessed on July 6, 2011.

Sengupta, S. 2007. "A Bangladeshi army of housewives battle tuberculosis." *New York Times.* April 5. http://www.nytimes.com/ 2007/04/05/world/asia/05iht-bangla.1.5156156.html. Accessed on June 30, 2011.

Sharma, B.V. 2002. Community contribution to TB care: an Asian perspective. Geneva: World Health Organization.

Sherzad, A.B. 2008. Health seeking behavior of smear positive tuberculosis patients receiving treatment from BRAC TB Centers in urban Dhaka. Master's thesis, James P. Grant School of Public Health, BRAC University.

Smiling Sun Franchise Program Website. "About us." http://www. smilingsunhealth.com/Default.aspx 2009. Accessed July 1, 2011.

Smillie, I. 1997. Words and Deeds: BRAC at 25. Dhaka: BRAC.

Smillie, I. 2009. Freedom from want: the remarkable success story of BRAC, the global grassroots organization that's winning the fight against poverty. Sterling: Kumarian Press.

Standing, H., Chowdhury, A.M.R. 2008. Producing effective knowledge agents in a pluralistic environment: what future for community health workers? *Social Science and Medicine.* 66, 2096-2107.

Stop TB Website. "2007 Award Winners." 2011. http://www.stoptb.org/global/awards/kochon/awardees/2007.asp. Accessed on June 30, 2011.

TB Reider. 2010. Interventions for TB Control and Elimination. Slideshow. Updated September 29, 2010. http://www.tbrieder.org/interventions/interventions.html. Accessed July 19, 2011.

The Economist. 2010. BRAC in Business. *The Economist.* Feb 18, 2010. http://www.economist.com/node/15546464/print. Accessed on July 1, 2011.

Transparency International Bangladesh. Corruption Perception Index. 2010. October 26. http://www.ti-bangladesh.org/index.php?page_id=216. Accessed on July 1, 2011.

UNICEF. 2011. Goals for children and development in the 1990s. Information and Publications. http://www.unicef.org/wsc/goals.htm#Basicx. Accessed on July 6, 2011.

Urmee, S. 2011. Update on Smiling Sun Franchise Program TB control activities. At the Urban DOTS Workshop. February 9. Dhaka.

Uvin, P., Miller, D. 1996. Paths to scaling up: alternative strategies for local nongovernmental organizations. *Human organization*. 55; 344-354.

Walt, V. 2009. Report: Attacks on aid workers on the rise. *Time*. April 9. http://www. time.com/time/world/article/0,8599,1890311,00.html. Accessed on July 1, 2011.

Whitworth, J. 2003. World Health Organization/International Society of Hypertension statement on management of hypertension. *Journal of Hypertension*. 21; 1983-1992.

World Bank. World Development Indicators Database. Data from 2006 and 2008. http://ddp-ext.worldbank.org/ext/ddpreports/ ViewSharedReport?&CF=& REPORT_ID=10200&REQUEST_TYPE=VIEWADVANCED&HF=N&WSP=N. Accessed on July 1, 2011.

World Health Organization, Afghanistan. About TB in Afghanistan. http://www .emro.who.int/afghanistan/programmes_stb_cf_tb_burden.htm. Accessed on July 1, 2011.

World Health Organization, Country Office for Bangladesh. 2010. Fifth Joint monitoring mission of the Bangladesh National Tuberculosis Control Programme. World Health Organization. BAN-TUB-45.

World Health Organization. 2006. The world health report 2006: working together for health. Geneva: World Health Organization. http://www.who.int/whr/2006/ whr06_en.pdf. Accessed on July 1, 2011.

World Health Organization. 2007. Prevention of cardiovascular disease: guidelines for risk assessment and management of cardiovascular risk. World Health Organization.

World Health Organization. 2009. Afghanistan: Global Health Observatory. http://www.who.int/countries/afg/en/. Accessed on July 1, 2011.

World Health Organization. 2010. Treatment of tuberculosis guidelines. 4th ed. Geneva: World Health Organization. http://whqlibdoc.who.int/publications/ 2010/9789241547833_eng.pdf. Accessed on July 12, 2011.

World Health Organization. 2011. Guidelines for the programmatic management of drug-resistant tuberculosis—2011 update. Geneva: World Health Organization. http://whqlibdoc.who.int/publications/2011/9789241501583_eng.pdf. Accessed on July 12, 2011.

World Health Organization. 2011. "Tuberculosis and HIV." In *HIV*. http://www. who.int/hiv/topics/tb/en/. Accessed on July 12, 2011.

World Health Organization. 2011. Sixty-four World Health Assembly closes after passing multiple reforms. 24 May. http://www.who.int/mediacentre/news/releases/2011/world_health_assembly_20110524/en/index.html. Accessed on July 1, 2011.

World Health Organization. 2011. Towards universal access to diagnosis and treatment of multidrug-resistant and extensively drug-resistant tuberculosis by 2015: WHO progress report. Geneva: World Health Organization.

World Health Organization. Bangladesh Country Page. http://www.whoban.org/hiv_aids.html. Accessed on July 1, 2011.

World Health Organization. Country statistics. 2007. http://apps.who.int/ ghodata/? vid=4200&theme=country. Accessed on July 1, 2011.

Yesudian Hannah Monica. 2007. Assessment of Tuberculosis Control Activities in Workplaces in Chittagong and in Dhaka, Bangladesh. World Health Organization. http://www.stoptb.org/countries/tbteam/docs/1_17_107_BAN-TUB-05_work%20places_Dec07.pdf. Accessed on July 1, 2011.

Zaman, K., Rahim, Z., Yunus, M., Arifeen, S., Baqui, A. 2005. Drug resistance of Mycobacterium tuberculosis in selected urban and rural areas in Bangladesh. *Scandinavian Journal of Infectious Diseases.* 37; 21-26.

Index

13130

13177

13130

Heath